Frontiers in Arthritis

(Volume 1)

Management of Osteoarthritis - A Holistic View

Edited by

Ashish Anand

GV Montgomery Veteran Affairs Medical Center,
Jackson, Mississippi,
USA
Department of Orthopedic Surgery,
University of Mississippi Medical Center,
Jackson, Mississippi,
USA

Frontiers in Arthritis

Management of Arthritis-A Holistic View

Volume # 1

Editor: Ashish Anand

eISSN (Online): 2468-6670

ISSN (Print): 2468-6662

eISBN (Online): 978-1-68108-351-3

ISBN (Print): 978-1-68108-352-0

First published in 2017.

advertisements or ideas contained in the Work.

Limitation of Liability:

In no event will Bentham Science Publishers, its staff, editors and/or authors, be liable for any damages, including, without limitation, special, incidental and/or consequential damages and/or damages for lost data and/or profits arising out of (whether directly or indirectly) the use or inability to use the Work. The entire liability of Bentham Science Publishers shall be limited to the amount actually paid by you for the Work.

General:

1. Any dispute or claim arising out of or in connection with this License Agreement or the Work (including non-contractual disputes or claims) will be governed by and construed in accordance with the laws of the U.A.E. as applied in the Emirate of Dubai. Each party agrees that the courts of the Emirate of Dubai shall have exclusive jurisdiction to settle any dispute or claim arising out of or in connection with this License Agreement or the Work (including non-contractual disputes or claims).

2. Your rights under this License Agreement will automatically terminate without notice and without the need for a court order if at any point you breach any terms of this License Agreement. In no event will any delay or failure by Bentham Science Publishers in enforcing your compliance with this License Agreement constitute a waiver of any of its rights.

3. You acknowledge that you have read this License Agreement, and agree to be bound by its terms and conditions. To the extent that any other terms and conditions presented on any website of Bentham Science Publishers conflict with, or are inconsistent with, the terms and conditions set out in this License Agreement, you acknowledge that the terms and conditions set out in this License Agreement shall prevail.

Bentham Science Publishers Ltd.
Executive Suite Y - 2
PO Box 7917, Saif Zone
Sharjah, U.A.E.
Email: subscriptions@benthamscience.org

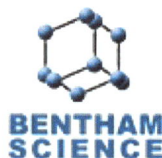

BENTHAM SCIENCE

CONTENTS

FOREWORD

Osteoarthritis is known enigma for Orthopedic Surgeons and it continues to be amongst the most important cause of chronic pain and disability. It is estimated that around 6 billion dollars/year are spent alone on management of this epidemic.

The purpose of this monograph is to offer the reader treatment options available for the management of osteoarthritis of knee and hip. If one reviews the current spectrum of literature available to, it becomes clear that there is a large body of literature in which the patient has to sort through with varying degree of scientific evidence, making anyone embarking on this Journey a difficult and conducing one. This Monograph provides an in depth analysis of the Pathology, Role of Nutrition and Exercise in treatment of arthritis there by offering a unique perspective to the Reader.

The book also provides insights into Role of injectables such as Platelet rich plasma and Viscosupplementation and elaborates on the Role of Amniofix- stem cells from the Amnion and Chorion in the treatment of Osteoarthritis. Finally, the book presents a number of surgical options for the reader that have had an established place for decades in the field of surgical arthritis such as Osteotomy, Arthroscopy and Replacement surgery.

Dr. Ashish Anand, MD has done a commendable Job in editing the manuscript. This book is a good read for Medical students, residents in training and the busy practitioner.

Khaled J. Saleh
President Orthopaedic Education

PREFACE

The book contains eight chapters with initial ones focusing on pathology behind osteoarthritis, Role of Nutrition in management of Osteoarthritis and Role of exercise in Management of Osteoarthritis. All of them point and educate the reader/clinician on their important role in pathogenesis as well as prevention of osteoarthritis. The Reader is encouraged to incorporate Nutrition and Exercise management in his Clinical practice.

The next chapter tells us about the Role of Viscosupplementation and Platelet Rich Plasma(PRP) in management of osteoarthritis and what the current clinical evidence is for the above two modalities.

Chapter 5 is an interesting chapter on Amniofix, which is relatively unheard of. Amniofix is an allograft tissue obtained from a Human baby and contains growth factors which have the potential for treating osteoarthritis pain when everything has failed and the patient is not interested in surgery. It may even possibly reverse the early damaging changes to the Cartilage. As time goes by, I am sure one will hear a lot about this "Novel" approach.

The second last section deals with surgical aspects of treatment of arthritis of knee in which the book dwells on the role of Arthroscopy with Cartilage Surgery, role of Osteotomy around the knee, and Current Concepts in Total Knee Replacement.

The last section deals with surgical management of arthritis of Hip-namely Role of Arthroscopy with Cartilage Surgery as well as Current Concepts in Total hip replacement.

It is my sincere hope that this book will stimulate the minds of the busy clinicians to read more about the subject and possibly also add some new tools to their armamentarium to give their patients the best possible treatment.

Ashish Anand
GV Montgomery Veteran
Affairs Medical Center, Jackson,
Mississippi, USA
Department of Orthopedic Surgery
University of Mississippi Medical Center
Jackson, Mississippi
USA

ACKNOWLEDGEMENTS

I always used to wonder what does work of an editor involve? All my questions were answered as I worked diligently during the preparation of this monograph. It gave me sleepless nights so that I could stick to the schedule given to me by the publishers. Interacting with the various authors and then editing their work was an excellent learning experience. I would like to thank all the authors who spent there valuable time in preparing the manuscripts and sticking to my schedule. All of us enjoyed writing this book and we sincerely hope that the reader gets the same pleasure and adds something more to his knowledge while reading this book.

I am indebted to my parents for instilling the values of hard work, perseverance and commitment as all these qualities served me in good stead during the preparation of this manuscript. I would like to thank my wife Varsha for constantly nudging me to go above and beyond. Finally, I would like to thank my two lovely daughters Advikaa and Vahita for helping me out with computer glitches and sparing me valuable time without which this book would not have seen light of the day.

Ashish Anand
GV Montgomery Veteran
Affairs Medical Center, Jackson,
Mississippi, USA
Department of Orthopedic Surgery
University of Mississippi Medical Center
Jackson, Mississippi
USA

List of Contributors

Ashish Anand	Staff Orthopedic Surgeon, GV Montgomery Medical Center, Jackson, Mississippi USA and Assistant Professor(Adj), Department of Orthopedic Surgery. University of Mississippi Medical Center, Jackson, Mississippi, USA
Ashley L. Artese	Department of Nutrition, Food and Exercise Sciences, Florida State University, Tallahassee, FL, USA
Avijit Sharma	OSU Sports Medicine and Cartilage Restoration Program, The Ohio State University Wexner Medical Center, Columbus, Ohio, USA
Bahram H. Arjmandi	Department of Nutrition, Food and Exercise Sciences, Florida State University, Tallahassee, FL, USA. Center for Advancing Exercise and Nutrition Research on Aging, Florida State University, Tallahassee, FL, USA
Brandon F. Grubbs	Department of Nutrition, Food and Exercise Sciences, Florida State University, Tallahassee, FL, USA
B. Zampogna	Department of Orthopaedic and Trauma Surgery, Campus Biomedico University of Rome, Via Alvaro del Portillo 200, Rome, Italy
Carmen Frias Kletecka	Department of Pathology, 1901 Perdido Street, Box P5-1, New Orleans, LA 70112, USA
Christina Leta	Department of Nutrition, Food and Exercise Sciences, Florida State University, Tallahassee, FL, USA
Daniel L. Murphy	University of Mississippi Medical Center, Jackson, MS
David C. Flanigan	OSU Sports Medicine and Cartilage Restoration Program, The Ohio State University Wexner Medical Center, Columbus, Ohio, USA
Fiona Blanco-Kelly	Fundación Jiménez Díaz University Hospital, Quirón Salud, Madrid, Spain
JV Srinivas	Clinical Director Consultant Orthopedic Surgeon, Fortis Hospital, Bannerghatta road, Bangalore, India
Lauren A. Foy	ATC University of Florida, FL, USA
Mark F. Sommerfeldt	OSU Sports Medicine and Cartilage Restoration Program, The Ohio State University Wexner Medical Center, Columbus, Ohio, USA
Maurizio Montalti	Laboratorio di Tecnologia Medica, Istituto Ortopedico Rizzoli, Bologna, Italy.
Mohan Puttaswamy	Consultant Orthopedic Surgeon, Fortis Hospital, Bannerghatta road, Bangalore, India
Narayan Hulse	Additional Director of Orthopaedics, Fortis Hospital, Banneragatta Road, Bengaluru, India

N. Maffulli Centre for Sports and Exercise Medicine, Barts and The London School of Medicine and Dentistry, Mile End Hospital, 275 Bancroft Road, London E1 4DG, England
Department of Musculoskeletal Disorders, Faculty of Medicine and Surgery, University of Salerno, 84081 Baronissi, Salerno, Italy

R. Papalia Department of Orthopaedic and Trauma Surgery, Campus Biomedico University of Rome, Via Alvaro del Portillo 200, Rome, Italy

R. Zini Department of Orthopaedic and Trauma Surgery, Villa Maria Cecilia Hospital, GVM Care & Research, Via Corriera 1, 48010 Cotignola, Ravenna, Italy

Saverio Affatato Laboratorio di Tecnologia Medica, Istituto Ortopedico Rizzoli, Bologna, Italy

Shirin Hooshmand School of Exercise and Nutritional Sciences, San Diego State University, San Diego, CA, USA

Víctor Vaquerizo Príncipe de Asturias University Hospital, Alcalá de Henares, Madrid, Spain

V. Denaro Department of Orthopaedic and Trauma Surgery, Campus Biomedico University of Rome, Via Alvaro del Portillo 200, Rome, Italy

DEDICATION

Dedicated to my brother, Rishi Anand.

Frontiers in Arthritis

CHAPTER 1

Pathology of Osteoarthritis

Carmen Frias Kletecka[*]

Louisiana State University Health Sciences Center, Department of Genetics, New Orleans, LA 70112, USA

Abstract: The pathology of osteoarthritis is extremely complex and multifactorial. Recent technological advances have allowed the identification of specific genes and genetic alterations which have helped to elucidate some intricacies involved in the molecular basis of disease development and progression. Known factors and key recent discoveries in pathogenesis, plus typical gross and histologic pathologic findings are described in this chapter.

Keywords: Degenerative joint disease, Gene, Genetic, Gross, Histology, Microscopic, Molecular, Morphology, Osteoarthritis, Pathology.

INTRODUCTION

Osteoarthritis (OA), also known as degenerative joint disease, is characterized by the progressive degradation of articular cartilage causing loss of function as a shock absorber [1]. The term OA was introduced by Archibald E. Garrod, an English physician in the 1890s [2]. The characteristic features of OA include initial softening, splitting, and fragmentation of articular cartilage followed by sclerosis of the bone underlying the articular surface cartilage (subchondral bone), bone cysts, and bony outgrowths at the joint margins (osteophytes) [3].

ETIOLOGY/PATHOGENESIS

OA is a multifactorial disease with a complex pathogenesis involving both environmental and genetic factors. The molecular basis of disease development

---

[*] **Corresponding author Carmen Frias Kletecka:** Louisiana State University Health Sciences Center, Department of Genetics, New Orleans, LA 70112, USA; Tel: 504-566-8571; Fax: 504-566-8454; E-mail: mfrias@lsuhsc.edu

Ashish Anand (Ed.)

and progression encompasses chondrocyte injury, repair, and ultimately, death. Chondrocyte injury elicits an inflammatory response and lymphocyte production of pro-inflammatory mediators, including TNF and IL-B. OA chondrocytes produce IL-1, inducing the expression of MMPs, and other catabolic enzymes. Pro-inflammatory mediators and catabolic enzymes subsequently lead to cartilage destruction [6]. In most cases, OA results from aging and an unknown underlying cause. In a minority of cases, OA develops in young patients with a predisposing condition, such as a previous joint injury, congenital deformity, or systemic disease. Environmental factors include aging and biomechanical stress related to physical characteristics like body weight and joint stability. Genetic factors include both intrinsic genes and altered gene expression *via* epigenetic modifications. Family and epidemiological studies show that OA is associated with multiple genes and has a heritability component. Genome wide association studies identified specific genes associated with the development and progression of OA [4, 5]. Genome wide methylation studies suggest that DNA methylation plays a significant role regulating the inflammation in cartilage through epigenetic modifications and together with cytokines, growth factors and changes in matrix composition, are involved in the development of OA. One in particular reports hypomethylation leading to increased transcription of pro-inflammatory factors including TFF, IL-1 and IL-6. Furthermore, epigenetic regulation involving microRNAs play a role in skeletal development and chondrogenesis [7, 8].

GROSS PATHOLOGY

The osteoarthritic articulating joint commonly displays cartilaginous outgrowths or osteophytes and loss of normal roundness. In the early stages of OA, hyaline cartilage on the articular surface is soft and granular. With disease progression, the articular cartilage sloughs off and is partially or completely lacking over weight bearing areas and remnants are usually present at the periphery. The underlying bone will have a polished, smooth appearance or eburnation in areas where it is in direct contact with another bone (Fig. **1**). The bony surface may have regenerative cartilage clusters where repair is taking place. Characteristic features seen on cross section include subchondral bone with a sclerotic appearance, subcortical cysts and wedge shaped necrosis (Fig. **2**). Subcortical cysts form when synovial fluid enters the subchondral bone space through small fractures on the bone surface. Multiple loose bodies may be present within the joint space [9 - 12].

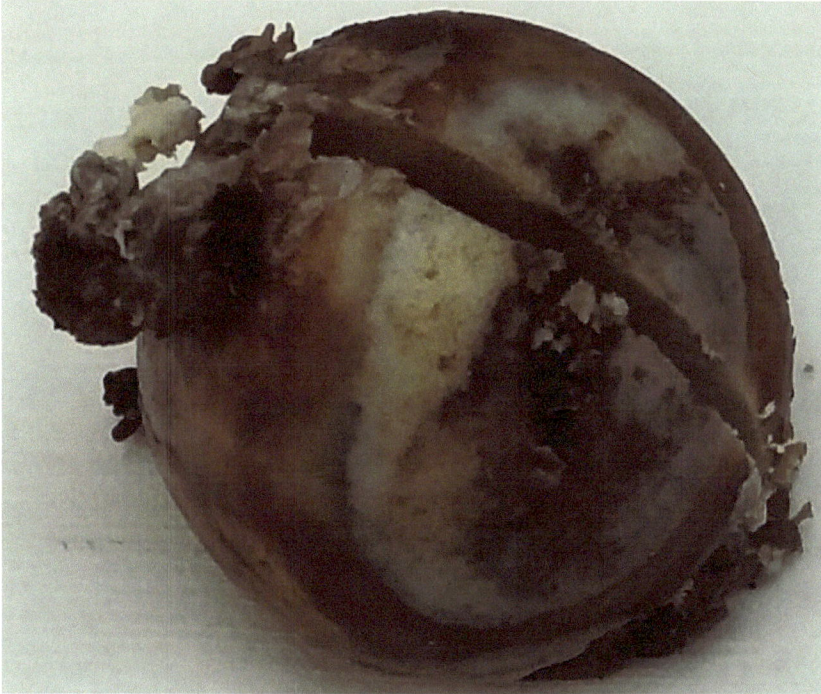

Fig. (1). Femoral head with osteoarthritis. The articular surface is eburnated and there are remnants of cartilage around the periphery *(Image courtesy of Reggie Thomasson, MD)*.

MICROSCOPIC PATHOLOGY

Injury and repair related changes are seen histologically within bone and cartilage tissue. As the superficial layers of cartilage and collagen degrade, vertical and horizontal fibrillation become apparent with subsequent matrix cracking. Cartilage repair or regeneration occurs both intrinsically and extrinsically. Intrinsic repair exists within the original articular hyaline cartilage as islands composed of chondrocyte clones within the matrix. Extrinsic repair presents as a highly cellular fibrocartilage with coarse and disorganized collagen overlying remnants of articular hyaline cartilage and at the joint margin (Fig. **3**).

Subchondral bone denuded of surface cartilage shows osteoblast proliferation and associated new bone formation, corresponding with areas of sclerosis seen grossly and on x-ray. Small fractures are commonly seen and may be associated with a subchondral cyst.

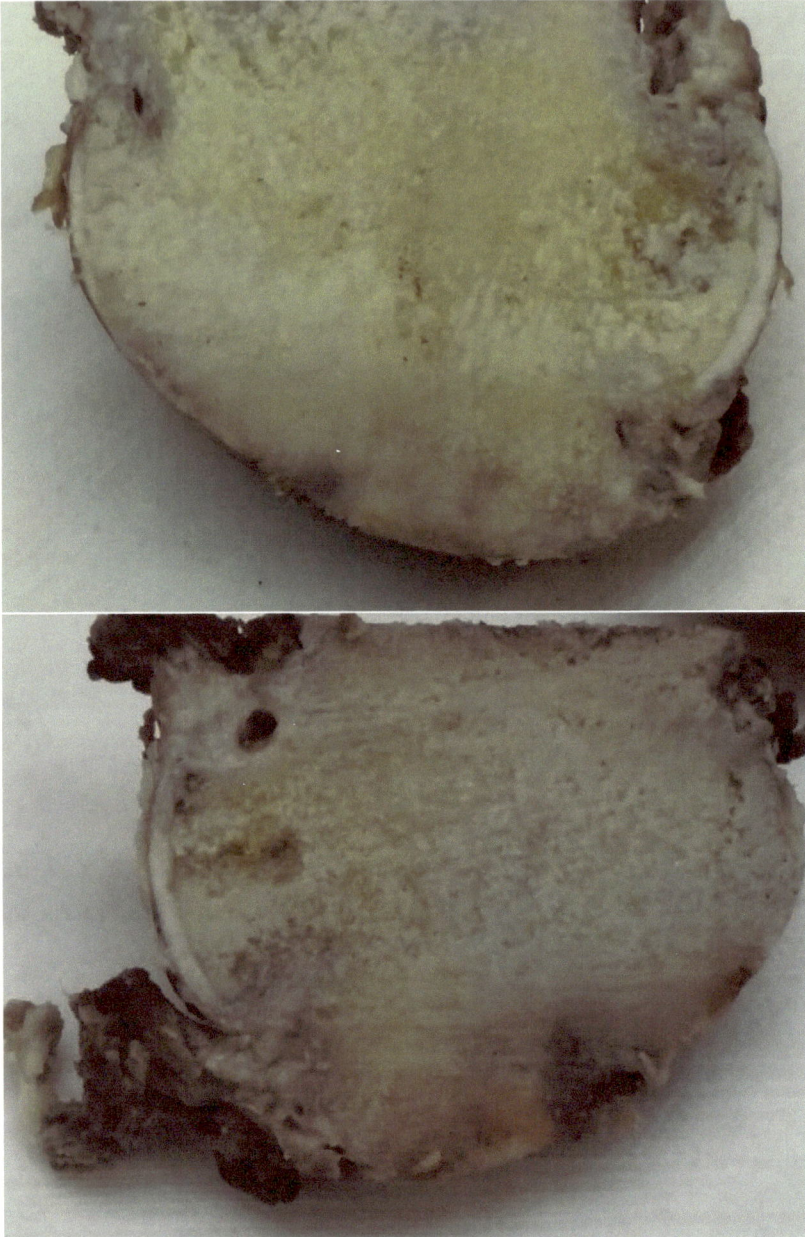

Fig. (2). Cross section of femoral head with osteoarthritis showing sclerotic subchondral bone, fracture and wedge necrosis *(Image courtesy of Joel France, DO).*

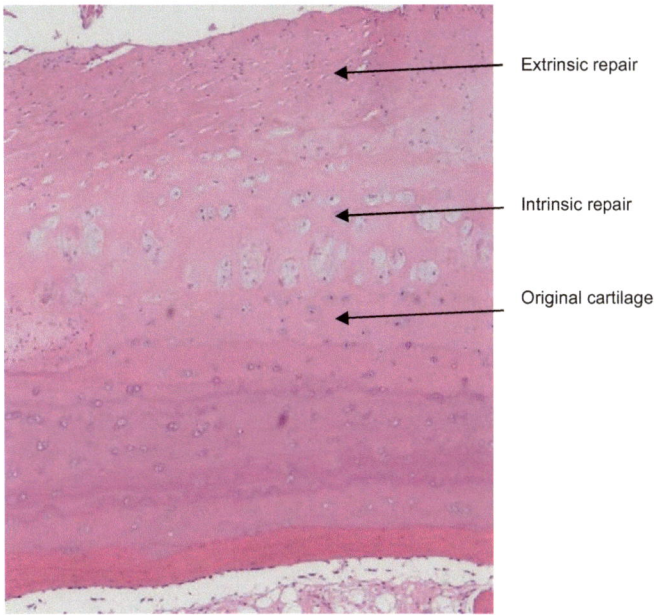

Fig. (3). Photomicrograph of cartilage with extrinsic and intrinsic repair.

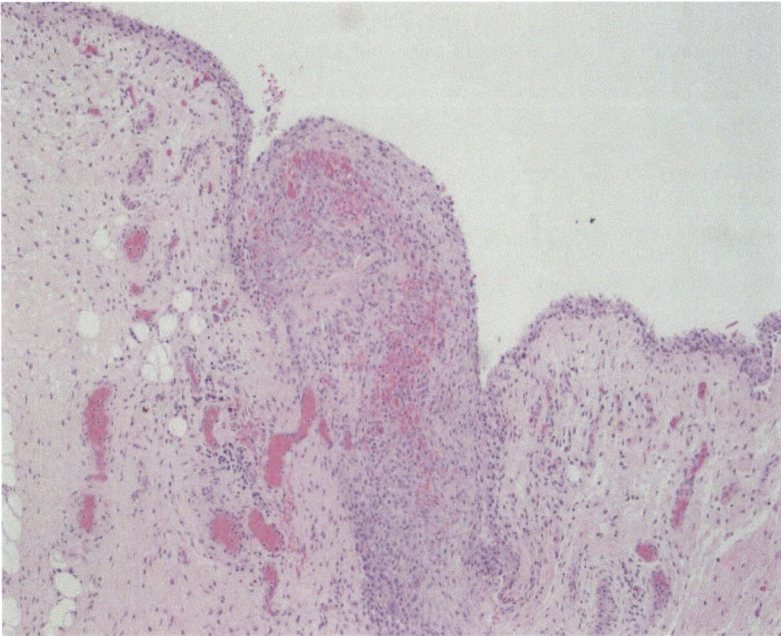

Fig. (4). Photomicrograph of synovium with hypertrophic and hyperplastic lining, stromal fibrosis, and chronic inflammation *(Image courtesy of Harry Porterfield, DO)*.

Synovium changes include stromal fibrosis of fibroadipose tissue, chronic inflammation, and both hyperplastic and hypertrophied lining (Fig. **4**).

Loose bodies typically have irregular, concentric calcified rings and cartilage replication.

CONFLICT OF INTEREST

The author confirms that the author has no conflict of interest to declare for this publication.

ACKNOWLEDGEMENTS

Declared none.

REFERENCES

[1]   Mankin HJ, Dorfman H, Lippiello L, Zarins A. Biochemical and metabolic abnormalities in articular cartilage from osteo-arthritic human hips. II. Correlation of morphology with biochemical and metabolic data. J Bone Joint Surg Am 1971; 53(3): 523-37.
[PMID: 5580011]

[2]   Garrod AE. A treatise on rheumatism and rheumatoid arthritis. Griffin 1890.

[3]   Dieppe P, Kirwan J. The localization of osteoarthritis. Br J Rheumatol 1994; 33(3): 201-3.
[http://dx.doi.org/10.1093/rheumatology/33.3.201] [PMID: 8156279]

[4]   Valdes AM, Spector TD. The contribution of genes to osteoarthritis. Rheum Dis Clin North Am 2008; 34(3): 581-603.
[http://dx.doi.org/10.1016/j.rdc.2008.04.008] [PMID: 18687274]

[5]   Warner SC, Valdes AM. The genetics of osteoarthritis: A review. J Fun Morp Kines 2016; 1(1): 140-53.
[http://dx.doi.org/10.3390/jfmk1010140]

[6]   Goldring MB, Goldring SR. Osteoarthritis. J Cell Physiol 2007; 213(3): 626-34.
[http://dx.doi.org/10.1002/jcp.21258] [PMID: 17786965]

[7]   Reynard LN. Analysis of genetics and DNA methylation in osteoarthritis: What have we learnt about the disease?. In Seminars in Cell and Developmental Biology 2016. Apr 26. Academic Press.

[8]   Roach HI, Aigner T. DNA methylation in osteoarthritic chondrocytes: a new molecular target. Osteoarthritis Cartilage 2007; 15(2): 128-37.
[http://dx.doi.org/10.1016/j.joca.2006.07.002] [PMID: 16908204]

[9]   Mills SE. Histology for pathologists. Lippincott Williams & Wilkins 2007; pp. 112-21.

[10]   The Noninflammatory Arthritides. Bullough PG, Ed. Orthopaedic Pathology. 5th ed., Philadelphia: Mosby 2010.

[11]   The Dysfunctional Joint. Bullough PG, Ed. Orthopaedic Pathology. 5th ed., Philadelphia: Mosby 2010.

[12]   Bullough PG. Joint diseases. In: Sternberg SS, Antonioli DA, Mills SE, Carter D, Oberman HA, Eds. Diagnostic Surgical Pathology. 3rd ed. Philadelphia, Pa: Lippincott Williams & Wilkins 1999; pp. 230-2.

CHAPTER 2

Exercise in the Prevention and Treatment of Osteoarthritis

Ashley L. Artese* and **Brandon F. Grubbs**

Department of Nutrition, Food and Exercise Sciences, Florida State University, Tallahassee, FL, USA

Abstract: Exercise can reduce the risk for osteoarthritis by aiding in the prevention of obesity, joint instability, and muscle weakness. It can also serve as an effective treatment by helping patients manage weight, improve muscular strength, decrease joint stiffness, improve range of motion, increase functionality, and reduce the risk for falls. Before starting an exercise program, patients should obtain a physician's consent and complete a thorough fitness assessment with an exercise specialist. The exercise program should be progressive, beginning with low-to-moderate intensity exercises followed by gradual increases in intensity. Low impact aerobic training and isometric or isotonic strength training are recommended modes of exercise for effective management of osteoarthritis symptoms. Yoga and tai chi provide low impact exercises and are considered effective therapy options for osteoarthritis symptom management. In addition, water-based exercise programs may improve adherence to an exercise program and be equally effective as land-based exercise for improving gait, functionality and pain. Since exercise adherence is the primary predictor of long-term outcomes in osteoarthritic patients, strategies to improve exercise adherence should be implemented.

Keywords: Aerobic, Exercise, Exercise adherence, Exercise prescription, Fall risk, Flexibility, Functionality, Isometric, Isotonic, Joint pain, Joint stiffness, Older adult, Osteoarthritis, Prevention, Strength, Tai chi, Treatment, Water exercise, Weight management, Yoga.

---

* **Corresponding author Ashley L. Artese:** Department of Nutrition, Food and Exercise Sciences, Florida State University, Tallahassee, FL, USA; Tel/Fax: (850) 644-1828/(850) 645-5000; E-mail: ala13b@my.fsu.edu

Ashish Anand (Ed.)

INTRODUCTION

Obesity, physical injury, joint instability, and muscle weakness are modifiable extrinsic risk factors associated with the development and progression of osteoarthritis. Obesity is a risk factor for several cardiovascular and metabolic diseases that plague more than one-third of U.S. adults and approximately 17% of American youth [1]. Gradual weight gain that leads to obesity can result from a combination of genetics, sedentary activity, and poor nutrition. Despite physical activity, aging adults reach their peak strength between the second and third decades in life. After 50 years of age, muscular strength declines at a rate of 12-15% per decade with even greater losses after 65 years [2]. Muscular power, the ability to generate force and velocity, is suggested to decline with greater magnitude and exceed losses in strength with age [3].

A lack of physical activity can accelerate declines in muscular performance and contribute to excessive weight gain. Higher body weight is associated with increased joint pain in older adults, and it has been estimated that the risk for developing osteoarthritis increases by 36% for every 5 kg increase in body weight [4]. Excess weight places additional load on the joint, which can lead to increased inflammation and structural changes in the joint and articular cartilage [5]. In addition to excess weight, a loss in both muscle mass and muscular strength, two important factors for joint movement, stability, and protection, are associated with joint degeneration and increased risk for osteoarthritis. These losses may be due to factors such as age-related sarcopenia, muscle-wasting diseases, and physical inactivity. Furthermore, obesity may contribute to these changes as intramuscular adipose tissue has been linked to losses in muscular strength and functional ability in older adults [6]. Both obesity and muscular weakness can affect movement and gait kinematics, which can cause the load-bearing portion of the joint to be shifted to areas that are not normally accustomed to the excess loading, resulting in cartilage degeneration and the progression of osteoarthritis [7]. The knees and the hips are the two most common joints affected by osteoarthritis as they are the joints which bear the greatest weight.

Comparatively, those who are physically active and participate in high impact sports are also at risk for osteoarthritis, as physical trauma can increase the disease's incidence [8]. Not only does damage to the joint affect the cartilage, but injury may lead to muscle weakness from disuse and weight gain from inactivity. Incorporating a safe and comprehensive exercise program into an individual's daily routine can help induce weight loss, prevent obesity, maintain muscular strength, and reduce injury, thus attenuating the development and symptoms of osteoarthritis.

Exercise Recommendations

The American College of Sports Medicine (ACSM), the largest sports medicine and exercise science organization in the world, has several position stands formulated from evidence of heavily scrutinized scientific literature. These position stands provide guidelines for appropriate physical activity intervention strategies for weight loss, weight regain, and health benefits. To avoid significant weight gain, ACSM recommends that adults engage in a minimum of 150 minutes per week of moderate intensity physical activity [9]. Overweight and obese adults can use the same recommendation to induce moderate weight loss; however, there is most likely a dose response relationship for exercise and weight reduction [9]. To achieve greater weight loss and prevent weight regain, ACSM recommends approximately 200 to 250 minutes of moderate intensity physical activity, which is equivalent to expending approximately 2,000 kcal, per week [9].

ACSM has also provided guidelines for physical activity for healthy older adults. These recommendations were developed based on evidence of the benefits of aerobic exercise and resistance training on health and functional capacity. For endurance, older adults should engage in moderate-intensity aerobic exercise accumulating at least 30 minutes of exercise time per day in bouts of at least 10 minutes to total 150-300 minutes per week. If working at a vigorous intensity, older adults should accumulate 20-30 minutes per day or more to total 75-150 minutes per week [10]. To determine the level of physical exertion, a 0 to 10 point scale is used where a score of 10 equals maximal physical exertion. Moderate intensity is a 5 to 6 and vigorous intensity is 7 to 8. Aerobic exercise modalities that do not exacerbate symptoms of orthopedic stress such as walking, cycling, and aquatics are recommended [10].

In addition to endurance training, ACSM recommends that older adults engage in at least 2 days per week of resistance training. This can be accomplished with the use of free weights or dumbbells, machines, ankle weights, or strengthening activities such as stair climbing. Exercisers should work between moderate (5-6) and vigorous (7-8) intensities [10]. Older adults participating in a strength program should do so with caution as there is risk for musculoskeletal injury. Using a progressive weight training program design that increases the exercise intensity gradually throughout the program can minimize this risk and optimize gains in strength. Resistance training may be optimal for obese older adults or those experiencing mobility impairment since minimal ambulation is required. While resistance training is not recommended as an effective strategy for weight loss, it does provide favorable changes in body composition that result in reductions in abdominal adipose tissue and increases in lean mass.

Treatment of Osteoarthritis

Osteoarthritic changes are most common in older adults. While no cure exists for osteoarthritis, the most effective strategy is to utilize interventions that target the disease's symptoms. Exercise has been shown to help osteoarthritic patients manage weight, improve muscular strength, decrease joint stiffness, improve range of motion, increase functionality, and reduce the risk for falls and fractures [11], which can ultimately lead to increased quality of life. Those who do not exercise are prone to accelerated degeneration at the joint along with more pain and inflammation [12]. *Exercise can delay the need for arthroplasty and sometimes avoid it all together.*

Pain is the most common symptom of osteoarthritis and this can be accompanied by joint stiffness, inflammatory swelling, instability, and muscle weakness. Together these symptoms can lead to physical limitations which develop into impairments of independent living for older adults. Activities of daily living such as walking, house-cleaning, gardening, and stair-climbing become challenging and may then require the assistance of an aid. Exercise can improve functionality by increasing muscular strength, range of motion, proprioception (sensing of body stimuli and awareness of body part position, equilibrium, and motion), and cardiovascular fitness. Although exercise can reduce the symptoms associated with osteoarthritis, exercise cannot influence the structural impact of the disease.

While exercise is beneficial, adherence to a regular exercise regimen in this population is often difficult because of joint pain, symptom exacerbation, fatigue, decreased stability and balance, and additional comorbidities experienced by these patients [11]. Therefore, initial exercise intensity, frequency, volume, mode, and the individual's disease status must be taken into account when implementing an exercise training program in order to manage pain and discomfort and to prevent further symptom exacerbation. Since adherence is the primary predictor of long-term outcomes from exercise in these patients [13], strategies to improve exercise adherence should be implemented. These strategies include emphasis on group or individual instructional settings instead of a home-based exercise program, patient education on the benefits of exercise and the pathogenesis of the disease, and self-efficacy enhancement through progressive programs that emphasize small short-term goals along with encouragement provided by the instructor [14].

Prior to beginning an exercise program, an initial physician screening should be completed to identify health risks or safety concerns that may need to be addressed before or in the exercise program design. Next, a physical assessment is necessary to evaluate fitness level and functional ability so that a suitable starting point for the exercise program can be determined. Consulting an exercise specialist or exercise physiologist for assistance in the design of a program will ensure that the plan is both safe and individualized to meet the fitness needs and goals of the patient. Moreover, important safety concerns such as exercise technique, supportive footwear, and rest time should be addressed (see Table **4** for workout safety suggestions). At the beginning of an exercise program, patients should proceed slowly by incorporating a few low-to-moderate intensity exercises and gradually progress from there. For those who are bedridden or have low function, it may be beneficial to begin with only flexibility exercises to decrease stiffness in the joints and increase range of motion. From there, strength or aerobic exercise performed lying down, seated in a chair, in the pool, or with resistance machines can be progressively incorporated.

Based on clinical evidence of strength and aerobic interventions on osteoarthritis symptomology, the American Geriatrics Society has provided the following training guidelines for people with osteoarthritic pain (Table **1**). For aerobic exercise, participants should train 20 to 30 minutes per day for approximately 2 to 5 days per week. Exercise intensity should be low to moderate at 40-60% of VO_2 max or maximum heart rate (HRmax) [14]. Suggested aerobic exercise modalities are cycling, swimming, or walking. Several strengthening programs have been evaluated (isokinetic, isotonic, or isometric) to assess their impact on pain and functional measures, but current evidence does not favor one method over another [15]. Therefore, recommendations have been made based on two of the more common methods of strength training, isotonic and isometric.

Isometric exercises utilize contractions where the working muscle does not noticeably change in length and the affected joint does not move. This might be the preferred method of strength training for those experiencing severe pain and discomfort in the joint since movement is limited. To improve isometric strength, participants should train daily completing 1-10 contractions at 40-60% of their maximal voluntary contraction per muscle group and hold each contraction for approximately 1-6 seconds [14]. Strengthening exercises can be completed with the use of free weights, machines, and ankle weights. As the hip and knee joints are the greatest weight-bearing joints, strengthening exercises should focus on the hip and knee extensors, as these are also the muscles important for walking, sitting, and standing.

Table 1. 2001 general exercise guidelines by the AGS panel on exercise and osteoarthritis.

	Frequency	Intensity	Volume
Flexibility: Static Stretching	1x/day Goal is 3-5 days/wk	Stretch until subjective sensation of discomfort	1 stretch per major muscle group. Hold each stretch 5-15 sec Progress to 3-5 stretches per major muscle group for 20-30 sec
Strength: Isometric	Daily	Low-Moderate: 40-60% MVC	1-10 submaximal contractions per each major muscle group
Strength: Isotonic	2-3 days/wk	Low: 40% 1RM Moderate: 40-60% 1RM High: > 60% 1RM	10-15 repetitions 8-10 repetitions 6-8 repetitions
Endurance: Aerobic	3-5 days/wk	Low-Moderate: 40%-60% HRmax	Accumulate 20-30 min/day

Recreated from American Geriatrics Society Panel on Exercise and Osteoarthritis 2001. 1RM= 1 repetition max; MVC= maximal voluntary contraction; HRmax= maximal heart rate (220-age in years).

Isotonic contractions are combinations of concentric and eccentric movement with a non-changing application of force (traditional resistance training). For isotonic strength training, participants should exercise 2 to 3 days per week. After an initial 1 repetition maximum (1RM) assessment, participants should begin lifting at low intensity (40% 1RM) and complete approximately 10-15 repetitions per exercise. For moderate intensity, increase the load to 40-60% of 1RM and complete approximately 8-10 repetitions. For high intensity, the load should be greater than 60% 1RM and approximately 6-8 repetitions should be completed per exercise. Table **2** provides a list of exercises that can improve strength of the major muscle groups of the lower limbs.

Thus far, no evidence suggests one training method (aerobic *vs* strength) is more effective than the other, but rather the use of both might be the best strategy to address the range of impairments associated with osteoarthritis [13].

Table 2. Lower body strengthening exercises for the osteoarthritis patient.

Exercise	Exercise Description
Seated Leg Extension	1. Start seated in a chair with the legs bent at a 90° angle. 2. Extend one leg and hold for approximately 5-6 seconds. 3. Slowly lower leg back to the floor. 4. Relax and repeat for several repetitions before moving to the other side.
Quadriceps Flex	1. Start either lying down or standing. 2. Flex the quadriceps of one leg and hold for approximately 5-6 seconds. 3. Relax for 2-3 seconds and repeat.
Sit-to-Stand	1. This exercise requires a chair without wheels. 2. Sit in the middle of the chair and cross the arms over the chest while placing each hand on the opposite shoulder. 3. Keeping the feet flat on the floor, a straight back, and looking forward, rise from the chair to a standing position. 4. Slowly return to the seated position. 5. If extra support is needed, use hands or chair arms for assistance. *Increase intensity by holding a dumbbell close to the chest.
Gluteal Squeeze	1. Start lying down, standing, or seated. 2. Squeeze the gluteal muscles and hold for approximately 5-6 seconds. 3. Relax for 2-3 seconds and repeat.

(Table 2) contd.....

Exercise	Exercise Description
Stair-Climb	1. Ascend a flight of stairs as if simply traveling to the second floor of an office building. Work at a casual pace and use the hand rail for support if needed. 2. Stair dissention may also be helpful as the eccentric component to this exercise requires control and balance. *Increase intensity by carrying dumbbells in each hand or wearing a weighted vest.
Calf Raises	1. Start in a standing position with feet hip-width apart. 2. Slowly raise the heels off the ground while allowing the body to slightly lean forward to keep balance. Use a nearby stationary object like a counter top to help with balance as needed. 3. Keep a straight back and continue to rise until the body weight is on the balls of the feet. Hold this position briefly. 4. Inhale and slowly return your heels back to the floor. * Increase intensity by holding dumbbells by the sides of the body.
Standing Knee Flexion	1. Start in a standing position and use a counter top for balance. 2. Flex one leg to raise the heel until the knee is bent at 45°. Hold for 5-6 seconds. 3. Slowly return the foot to the floor. 4. Rest for 2-3 seconds and repeat. *Progressively increase the bend in the knee to include a greater range of motion. Next, adding ankle weights (3-5 lbs) can increase the resistance.
Knee Raise	1. Start standing with the hands placed on a nearby counter top for support. 2. Raise one knee upward until it is halfway to the hip. Maintain a strait back throughout the exercise. 3. Hold this position for approximately 5-6 seconds. 4. Slowly return the foot to the floor. 5. Rest 2-3 seconds and repeat.

Water-Based Exercise

While land-based exercise has been shown to improve disease status and progression, pain, and functional movement, it still may be a challenging activity for some patients due to pain and discomfort in the joint. An alternative method may be water-based exercise. Not only does the buoyancy of water help reduce stress and load on the joints, but it also allows patients to perform movements they would not normally be able to perform on land. Exercising in the water also helps prevent overheating and elicits lower blood pressures and heart rates at comparable land intensities. Water-based exercises are suggested to be just as effective as land-based exercise for the improvement of gait, functionality, and exercise adherence in knee osteoarthritis patients in addition to reducing joint pain [16]. While more research is needed to determine the effectiveness of water-based exercise along with appropriate program frequency, intensity, and duration for patients with both knee and hip osteoarthritis, a water-based exercise program may be a viable option, especially for those patients who are just beginning an exercise program, have increased joint pain, are carrying excess weight, or have balance and coordination concerns. Table **3** describes several exercises that can be performed in the water.

Table 3. Beginning water exercises for the osteoarthritis patient.

Exercise	Exercise Description
Pool Walking	1. Start in a standing position in shallow water with the feet flat on the floor, knees soft, abdominals engaged, and shoulders relaxed. 2. Walk across the pool floor, as if walking on land, placing the heel on the ground first and moving through to the ball of the foot. 3. Naturally move arms, placing the left arm forward when the right foot is stepping and right arm forward when the left leg is in front.
Knee Lifts	1. This exercise is similar to the water walking except an added knee lift is incorporated before each foot steps onto the floor. 2. Arms can move naturally, or press against the water with each step.
Hamstring Curls	1. Stand by the edge of the pool for support with both feet flat on the floor. 2. Bend the right knee and draw the right heel towards the right gluteal muscles. 3. Hold for 1-2 seconds and return to starting position. 4. Repeat 10-15 times on one side before continuing to the other side.
Lateral Walks	1. Travel laterally across the pool by stepping the right foot out to the side and then stepping the left foot in to meet the right. 2. Continue moving in the same direction for 10-15 repetitions or until the edge of the pool is reached. 3. Try to keep the feet facing forward throughout the exercise. 4. Repeat leading with the left leg.
Pool Squats	1. Stand facing the edge of the pool for support if needed with both feet flat on the floor, hips-distance width apart. 2. Slowly bend at the knees and hip to lower the hips down and back as if you are sitting in a chair. 3. Try to keep the back straight throughout the movement. 4. Hold at the bottom for 1-2 seconds and return to starting position. *Complete this exercise on one leg to increase the difficulty.
Calf Raises	1. Stand facing the edge of the pool for support if needed with both feet flat on the floor, hips-distance width apart. 2. Slowly raise the heels off of the floor until the balls of the feet are supporting the body weight. 3. Hold for 1-2 seconds and return to starting position.

(Table 3) contd.....

Exercise	Exercise Description
Gluteal Raises	1. Stand facing the edge of the pool for arm support if needed with both feet flat on the floor, hips-distance width apart. 2. Slowly lift and extend the right leg behind the body to a comfortable height. 3. Hold for 1-2 seconds and return to starting position. 4. Repeat 10-15 times before moving to the other side.
Single Leg Balance	1. Start with both feet flat on the floor. 2. Slowly lift the right leg off the floor and hold the position. 3. Maintain the position for 15-20 seconds and repeat on the other side.
Noodle Push-Downs	1. Place the middle of a pool noodle under the right foot. 2. Slowly press the right foot down until the noodle touches the floor. 3. Lift the foot off the floor by bending at the knee and hip until the thigh is parallel to the floor. 4. Repeat 10-15 times before switching to the left side.
Sea Horse	1. Straddle the pool noodle so that the back end is slightly higher than the front. 2. Travel around the pool by cycling legs and arms, focusing on range of motion.

Many patients might believe aquatic exercise is not an option for them because of limited pool access, facility membership cost, unfamiliarity with water classes, and mobility concerns. However, retirement communities and local organizations such as the YMCA and Senior Centers often have swimming pool facilities along with discounted memberships. Additionally, water classes of varying intensities may be offered by both facilities taught by certified instructors to provide participants with safe and effective instruction. For those with severe mobility impairment, pool lifts are often available and required to provide safe pool access.

Table 4. Workout safety suggestions for osteoarthritis patients.

Workout Safety Suggestions for Osteoarthritis Patients
• Wear supportive exercise or running shoes and replace approximately every 6 months. • Focus on technique for all exercises. Consult an exercise specialist or trainer for instruction on how to safely perform each exercise. • Always perform a 5-10 minute warm-up and a cool-down. • Perform static stretches at the end of the exercise session. • Stay hydrated by drinking water before, during, and after the exercise session. • Monitor pain during and after exercise. Excessive pain during exercise or continued pain following the exercise program may be a sign that the exercise intensity may need to be decreased.

Yoga and Tai Chi

Additional exercise alternatives for the management of osteoarthritis are the practice of yoga or tai chi, which are both mind-body practices. Hatha yoga is the physical practice of postures, known as asanas, combined with conscious breathing control to develop strength, flexibility, and balance. Tai chi is a low-impact form of Chinese martial arts that is practiced for both self-defense and health benefits including balance, strength, and stress relief. It consists of a sequence of martial arts movements, many derived from the natural movements of animals or birds, combined with deep breathing and meditation. Both may serve as beneficial treatments for reducing pain and joint stiffness while improving functionality, balance, and quality of life in osteoarthritis patients [17]. Yoga and tai chi classes may be offered through local YMCAs, Senior Centers, individual studios, retirement communities, and health and fitness facilities. For those with balance or mobility concerns, seated versions of these classes may also be available.

CONCLUSION

Regular exercise is an effective method for both the prevention and treatment of osteoarthritis. Aerobic and strength training along with water exercise, yoga, and tai chi are all considered feasible treatment options. Since adherence to an exercise program is the primary factor that influences long-term outcomes of osteoarthritis, it is important for the patient to participate in an activity that he or she enjoys and for healthcare providers or exercise specialists to provide guided instruction for these patients, consistently monitoring intensity, pain level, and physical exertion. In addition to one-on-one instruction, structured low-impact exercise classes specifically designed for older adults may be offered through local community centers and fitness facilities. Patients should consult a physician prior to beginning any exercise program to identify health risks and safety concerns so that an appropriate exercise plan can be designed.

ADDITIONAL RESOURCES

1. American College of Sports Medicine
   http://www.acsm.org
2. American Council on Exercise
   www.acefitness.org/acefit/exercise-library-main
3. Arthritis Foundation

http://www.arthritis.org
4. National Institute of Arthritis and Musculoskeletal and Skin Diseases.
   http://www.niams.nih.gov
5. National Institute of Senior Centers
   http://www.ncoa.org/national-institute-of-senior-centers
6. Silver Sneakers®
   https://www.silversneakers.com
7. Young Men's Christian Association (YMCA)
   http://www.ymca.net

CONFLICT OF INTEREST

The authors confirm that the author have no conflict of interest to declare for this publication.

ACKNOWLEDGEMENTS

Declared none.

REFERENCES

[1]   Ogden CL, Carroll MD, Kit BK, Flegal KM. Prevalence of childhood and adult obesity in the United States, 20112012. JAMA 2014; 311(8): 806-14.
      [http://dx.doi.org/10.1001/jama.2014.732] [PMID: 24570244]

[2]   Macaluso A, De Vito G. Muscle strength, power and adaptations to resistance training in older people. Eur J Appl Physiol 2004; 91(1): 450-72.
      [http://dx.doi.org/10.1007/s00421-003-0991-3] [PMID: 14639481]

[3]   Skelton DA, Greig CA, Davies JM, Young A. Strength, power and related functional ability of healthy people aged 6589 years. Age Ageing 1994; 23(5): 371-7.
      [http://dx.doi.org/10.1093/ageing/23.5.371] [PMID: 7825481]

[4]   Hart DJ, Spector TD. The relationship of obesity, fat distribution and osteoarthritis in women in the general population: the Chingford Study. J Rheumatol 1993; 20(2): 331-5.
      [PMID: 8474072]

[5]   Vincent KR, Vincent HK. Resistance exercise for knee osteoarthritis. PM R 2012; 4(5) (Suppl.): S45-52.
      [http://dx.doi.org/10.1016/j.pmrj.2012.01.019] [PMID: 22632702]

[6]   Marcus RL, Addison O, Dibble LE, Foreman KB, Morrell G, Lastayo P. Intramuscular adipose tissue, sarcopenia, and mobility function in older individuals. J Aging Res 2012; 2012: 629637.
      [http://dx.doi.org/10.1155/2012/629637] [PMID: 22500231]

[7]   Andriacchi TP, Mündermann A. The role of ambulatory mechanics in the initiation and progression of knee osteoarthritis. Curr Opin Rheumatol 2006; 18(5): 514-8.
[http://dx.doi.org/10.1097/01.bor.0000240365.16842.4e] [PMID: 16896293]

[8]   Lohmander LS, Englund PM, Dahl LL, Roos EM. The long-term consequence of anterior cruciate ligament and meniscus injuries: osteoarthritis. Am J Sports Med 2007; 35(10): 1756-69.
[http://dx.doi.org/10.1177/0363546507307396] [PMID: 17761605]

[9]   Donnelly JE, Blair SN, Jakicic JM, Manore MM, Rankin JW, Smith BK. American College of Sports Medicine Position Stand. Appropriate physical activity intervention strategies for weight loss and prevention of weight regain for adults. Med Sci Sports Exerc 2009; 41(2): 459-71.
[http://dx.doi.org/10.1249/MSS.0b013e3181949333] [PMID: 19127177]

[10]   Chodzko-Zajko WJ, Proctor DN, Fiatarone Singh MA, *et al.* American College of Sports Medicine position stand. Exercise and physical activity for older adults. Med Sci Sports Exerc 2009; 41(7): 1510-30.
[http://dx.doi.org/10.1249/MSS.0b013e3181a0c95c] [PMID: 19516148]

[11]   Marks R, Allegrante JP. Chronic osteoarthritis and adherence to exercise: a review of the literature. J Aging Phys Act 2005; 13(4): 434-60.
[http://dx.doi.org/10.1123/japa.13.4.434] [PMID: 16301755]

[12]   Hoffman DF. Arthritis and exercise. Prim Care 1993; 20(4): 895-910.
[PMID: 8310087]

[13]   Roddy E, Zhang W, Doherty M, *et al.* Evidence-based recommendations for the role of exercise in the management of osteoarthritis of the hip or kneethe MOVE consensus. Rheumatology (Oxford) 2005; 44(1): 67-73.
[http://dx.doi.org/10.1093/rheumatology/keh399] [PMID: 15353613]

[14]   Bennell KL, Hinman RS. A review of the clinical evidence for exercise in osteoarthritis of the hip and knee. J Sci Med Sport. Sports Medicine Australia 2011; 14(1): 4-9.
[http://dx.doi.org/10.1016/j.jsams.2010.08.002]

[15]   Pelland L, Brosseau L, Wells G, *et al.* Efficacy of strengthening exercises for osteoarthritis (part 1): a meta-analysis. Phys Ther Rev 2004; 9(2): 77-108.
[http://dx.doi.org/10.1179/108331904225005052]

[16]   Silva LE, Valim V, Pessanha AP, *et al.* Hydrotherapy *versus* conventional land-based exercise for the management of patients with osteoarthritis of the knee: a randomized clinical trial. Phys Ther 2008; 88(1): 12-21.
[http://dx.doi.org/10.2522/ptj.20060040] [PMID: 17986497]

[17]   Shengelia R, Parker SJ, Ballin M, George T, Reid MC. Complementary therapies for osteoarthritis: are they effective? Pain Manag Nurs 2013; 14(4): e274-88.
[http://dx.doi.org/10.1016/j.pmn.2012.01.001] [PMID: 24315281]

CHAPTER 3

Nutritional Impacts on Joint Health

Shirin Hooshmand[1], Christina Leta[2] and Bahram H. Arjmandi[2,3,*]

[1] *School of Exercise and Nutritional Sciences, San Diego State University, San Diego, CA*

[2] *Department of Nutrition, Food and Exercise Sciences, Florida State University, Tallahassee, FL*

[3] *Center for Advancing Exercise and Nutrition Research on Aging, Florida State University, Tallahassee, FL*

Abstract: Osteoarthritis is a common cause of musculoskeletal disability among the elderly. This can place burdens on society as this becomes more problematic for health care professionals to treat. For years, the management of osteoarthritic symptoms has been limited through the use of non-steroidal. Anti-inflammatory drugs (NSAID) for relief of pain and other debilitating symptoms. Since NSAIDs can cause other adverse side effects, nutritional supplements are being promoted as aids for preventing and reducing symptoms that relate to osteoarthritis without the development of adverse side effects. This chapter reviews the background of osteoarthritis as a degenerative joint disease while also looking at animal studies and human clinical trials that evaluate the effects of various nutritional supplements on joint health.

Keywords: Boron, Chondroitin sulfate, Curcumin, Dietary supplements, Dimethyl sulfoxide, Functional foods, Glucosamine sulfate, Inflammation, Joints, Magnesium, Nutrients, Omega-3, Osteoarthritis, Resveratrol, Soy, Vitamin E.

INTRODUCTION

Osteoarthritis (OA), known as degenerative arthritis, is the most common form of joint disease and is characterized by erosion of articular cartilage, thickening of subchondral bone and osteophyte formation [1]. Articular cartilage is a highly

---

* **Corresponding author Bahram H. Arjmandi:** Department of Nutrition, Food and Exercise Sciences, 412 Sandels Building, Florida State University, Tallahassee, FL 32306; Tel: (850) 645-1517; Fax: (850) 645-5000; E-mail: barjmandi@fsu.edu

Ashish Anand (Ed.)

specialized connective tissue consisting of water, collagen and proteoglycan. The conformation of these components creates a stiff fiber-reinforced water gel with friction and shock-absorbing capacity. Joints that can be most affected by OA are of the knee, hips, hands, and spine. Symptoms of OA include but are not limited to localized pain that is worsened with activity and relieved by rest, stiffness and decreased range of motion [2, 3]. With advanced OA, weight bearing joints may give out and joints will develop bony enlargements. These bony knobs (nodes) will enlarge the finger joints creating a gnarled appearance. These nodes can take years to appear. OA will gradually worsen over time yet no cure is available. Cartilage degeneration is due to failure in the elastic restraint because of alterations in the structure of collagen. Degenerative conditions are also accompanied by local inflammatory components that may accelerate the joint destruction. The proteoglycan content in OA is gradually depleted, leading to an increase in water content and a loss of compressibility and shock absorption.

OA can be caused from previous joint injury, abnormal joint development, genetics, muscle weakness, joint instability and repetitive microtrauma. Two major risk factors for OA are increasing age, with most patients affected being 45 years and older, and increasing obesity [1]. However, staying active and maintaining a healthy weight through proper diet may help slow progression of the disease and help improve pain and joint function [4]. Conventional treatments, commonly prescribed pharmaceuticals, are available to those suffering from OA; however, adverse side effects are often associated with prescription medications. Non-steroidal anti-inflammatory drugs (NSAIDs) and analgesics can often relieve symptoms of OA but can cause peptic ulcers, hepatic or renal failure. While failing to prevent or delay the progression of the disease, NSAIDs may accelerate joint destruction when used as a long-term pain relief [3, 5]. The need to develop safer and more effective ways for treating OA is still needed. Other alternative approaches for therapeutic treatment are through natural, herbal, physical manipulation, holistic and nutritional techniques. Many substances that occur naturally within the body, may pose as a valuable treatment method for managing OA, as well as some functional foods, as these methods may present long-term pain relief as well as keeping the structural damage of the cartilage to a minimum. In most cases, a nutritional compound has only limited effects on its biological target and pertinent differences are reached over time through a buildup effect, in which case the benefits will add up day after day. In theory, chronic diseases like OA should benefit from nutrition, more so than acute diseases. The appeal of using nutrition coincides with ailment prevention. Long-term pharmacological interventions for OA are frequently associated with adverse side effects. Nutraceuticals, a term coined from 'nutrition' and 'pharmaceutical' and defined as a food or part of a food that provides *medicinal* or health benefits to prevent or treat a disease, and functional foods could provide an advantageous alternative because, by laws, they have to be devoid of adverse effects [6].

ROLE OF NATURAL SUPPLEMENTS FOR PREVENTION AND TREATMENT OF OSTEOARTHRITIS

Nutritional Supplements have been developed for individuals with OA and have become popular because these supplements can provide the natural components that are able to inhibit or enhance the biological mediators that are able to preserve the structure of the joint [7]. Nutraceuticals are functional ingredients that are sold as powders, pills, and other medicinal forms that are not generally associated with food.

Glucosamine Sulfate and Chondroitin Sulfate

Glucosamine Sulfate is found both in the human body, produced from glucose, as well as found in nature among shellfish, and commonly used to treat arthritis. Articular cartilage contains a group of large protein molecules called proteoglycans. These are the proteins that give cartilage its strength and flexibility [3]. Glucosamine is an important precursor in the biosynthesis of many connective tissue macromolecules such as hyaluronic acid, glycosaminoglycan's (GAGs), glycolipids, and glycoproteins.

Glucosamine and Chondroitin are among the most popular OA supplements. Gaby suggests that glucosamine supplements may be an effective treatment for OA [3]. Articular pain, joint tenderness, swelling, and range of motion greatly improved in clinical trial groups that received glucosamine treatment compared to the counterpart group that only received a placebo [8]. This suggests that glucosamine supplements may slow the progression of the disease unlike current pharmaceuticals. Many individuals suffering from OA will take acetaminophen or NSAIDs for pain relief, which can eventually cause stomach ulcers and cartilage degradation after long-term use. There have also been studies that have compared the efficacy of glucosamine supplement treatment to NSAIDs such as ibuprofen. Individuals who took 1,500 mg per day of glucosamine had improved pain relief compared to individuals taking 1,200 mg of ibuprofen per day [9]. Both of those groups had reduced pain symptoms but glucosamine supplements were trending to be more effective. There have been no adverse side effects associated with the use of glucosamine supplements as it is generally better tolerated than NSAIDs [9].

Chondroitin Sulfate consists of repeating chains of molecules called mucopolysaccharides. Chondroitin is classified as a type of glycosaminoglycan's that is rich in sulfur and related to glucosamine. Chondroitin Sulfate, found in the human body and also shark cartilage, is also a GAG found in articular cartilage. The articular cartilage is able to absorb large quantities of water because of its hydrophilic properties. The water absorption helps with handling the compressive forces that the cartilage will withstand [7].

Levels of chondroitin sulfate may be reduced in joint cartilage that is affected by OA and other forms of arthritis. Chondroitin sulfate supplements may help to restore joint function in individuals affected by OA. These effects may be similar with glucosamine sulfate supplements. Animal studies have indicated that chondroitin sulfate may promote healing of bone since the majority of GAG's found in bone consist of chondroitin sulfate.

Glucosamine sulfate and chondroitin sulfate have also being tested for efficacy when administered in combination to determine if the combined supplements could provide additional benefits over solitary supplementation. There is still only limited data regarding the effects of combined treatment on humans. However, when glucosamine sulfate and chondroitin sulfate are combined with hydrochloride (HCl), there was pain relief and improved function for patients suffering from OA in the knee [10].

Is glucosamine sulfate better than chondroitin sulfate at alleviating pain for those suffering from osteoarthritis? When glucosamine sulfate is given orally, it has been shown to be well absorbed. On the other hand, chondroitin sulfate is a larger molecule that is mainly hydrolyzed in the intestinal tract prior to being absorbed. With that said, the amount absorbed is understood to be small. If chondroitin sulfate is mainly broken down in the intestinal tract, then administering chondroitin sulfate is an expensive means to obtain precursor molecules. However, since glucosamine sulfate serves as a precursor molecule to chondroitin sulfate, administering glucosamine sulfate may be a less expensive method of increasing the content of chondroitin sulfate in the joint cartilage. Though, some believe that the small amount of chondroitin sulfate that is absorbed, gives beneficial effects that cannot be duplicated by glucosamine. Until further studies are conducted, the choice of which supplement to use is at the discretion of the individual [3, 9].

Vitamin E

The human body has an extensive antioxidant defense system. A number of smaller antioxidants play an important role where antioxidant enzymes are spares. The idea is that these smaller, micronutrient, antioxidants will provide additional defense against tissue injury when the enzymes (superoxide dismutase, catalase, and peroxidase) are overwhelmed. It is hypothesized that a diet rich in vitamin E (α-tocopherol), β-carotene (a vitamin A precursor), and vitamin C (ascorbate), might protect against age-related disorders [11]. Studies have shown either a decrease in pain at rest and during movement as well as increases in joint mobility with vitamin E supplementation when compared with a placebo or diclofenac, a NSAID. Though, the mechanism behind how vitamin E works with OA is unknown, vitamin E has been reported to have anti-inflammatory roles. Yet, vitamin E may inhibit the release of enzymes that are believed to play a role in the development of osteoarthritic joint damage [3, 11].

A study examining the North Indian geriatric population, found a strong correlation between plasma C-reactive protein (CRP) levels and synovial fluid interleukin-6 (IL-6) levels. IL-6 is one of the main regulators of CRP production that plays a role in the inflammatory process. Elevated IL-6 levels have been found to be associated with synovitis, an inflammation of the synovial membrane, and degeneration in individuals with OA. After taking vitamin E supplementation, there was no major reduction in plasma CRP or IL-6 levels [12]. Those who have OA and have a diet high in antioxidants will show a much slower rate of joint deterioration as compared to individuals who have a diet low in antioxidants. While some studies have shown beneficial evidence for incorporating Vitamin E, there is still no clear-cut recommendation for its use.

Boron

Boron is a trace element that, if its' intake is too little or too much, is harmful to human health. Although there is no recommended dietary allowances (RDA) or recommended daily intake (RDI) for boron consumption, ingestion of 1-10 mg daily is preferred. In terms of OA, the findings of an 8-week study suggested that taking 6 mg/day of sodium tetraborate, elemental boron, was more efficient than a placebo for reducing a patients' assessment of symptoms. However, a longer clinical trial is required to more thoroughly evaluate the benefits of boron for treating OA [3, 13].

Rex Newnham hypothesized that the lack of dietary boron would enhance the occurrence and severity of different forms of arthritis, or that supplementation with boron could aid in alleviating arthritic conditions. The hypothesis was based on self-experimentation of supplementing the diet with 6 mg/day of sodium tetraborate to alleviate arthritic pain; swelling and stiffness. Between 1976 and 1981, *about* 90,000 bottles of elemental boron were sold without advertising. Newnham presented the experiment to the Australian and New Zealand Association for the Advancement of Science in Auckland, New Zealand, in 1979, to show the concentration of boron in healthy femur heads compared to arthritic femur heads [3, 13].

Similar findings of lower boron concentrations in bone and synovial fluid in individuals with rheumatoid arthritis compared to those without rheumatoid arthritis have been observed. However, Australia later declared boron and its compounds to be poisonous in any concentration. The banning of boron for consumption is what led Newnham to gather scientific evidence to support the need for dietary boron. Newnham determined a relationship between arthritis and low boron exposure based on epidemiology. These findings suggest that global locations where boron intake is ≤ 1mg, reveals an occurrence of arthritis ranged from 20%-70%, where as other locations consuming 3 mg - 10 mg of boron portrayed lower instances of arthritis ranging from 0%-10% [3, 13].

Other findings that help support the beneficial need of boron for bone health come from surgeons that proclaim patients taking boron supplements will have much tougher bones, as the bones are more difficult to cut than bones of individuals who are not taking a boron supplementation. Clinical observations have also shown that boron supplements will accelerate the healing process to repair broken bones [3, 13].

Evidence over 30 years points towards the need for boron to help preserve healthy bones and joints. Epidemiological studies suggested that boron supplementation; in the amount found in some diets throughout the world can be effective for preventing and treating different forms of arthritis. Likewise, boron should not be considered a poison or a pharmaceutical agent because there are inadequate data to support either of the views. Further research is still needed to determine whether individuals with a diet high in boron can still benefit from boron supplementation. The average American can receive their daily amount of boron, about 1-2 mg, from fruits, vegetables and nuts. Boron has been shown to modulate bone and calcium metabolism that play a role in preserving bone mineral density (BMD). Also, boron has been reported to reduce the urinary excretion of calcium and magnesium, which positively influence bone and calcium metabolism [14]. Boron also has the capacity to increase estrogen levels and this may raise questions about any possible risk for cancer. However, as mentioned earlier there is a paucity of data to suggest that boron should be taken as a supplement [3, 13]. Nonetheless, if individuals consume a variety of plant based foods *e.g.* prunes, nuts, and legumes they should receive adequate amounts of boron [3, 13].

Magnesium

Several studies have examined the effect of magnesium supplementation on chondrocyte and cartilage integrity, as well as joint health. Magnesium has been shown to positively affect damaged chondrocyte and cartilage. Magnesium also has been shown to be beneficial when it is injected into the knee joint, improving the damaged joint and synovial fluid. The goal of treating OA is to reduce inflammation along with decreasing pain associated with the disease. Knee joints that were treated with the magnesium injection showed a decrease in knee joint width due to less inflammation. Magnesium injection into synovitis has also been shown to be less severe after the magnesium injection [15, 16].

When magnesium is in direct contact with the chondrocytes, the integrity of the chondrocyte improves while pain decreases yet the definitive role of magnesium treatments for OA are not currently apparent; hence further studies are needed to confirm its role in OA.

Omega-3 Fatty Acid

Omega-3 polyunsaturated fatty acids (PUFA) are found in flaxseeds, walnuts, fish oil, and soybeans. A diet high in omega-3 is associated with a lower occurrence of cardiovascular disease; having anti-arrhythmic, anti-thrombotic, anti-inflamma-tory, anti-hypertensive, and anti-hyperlipidemia effects. Supplementation with PUFA have been used in clinical trials to assess its beneficial functions for individuals with rheumatoid arthritis and it has been shown that the encapsulated fish oil reduces the number of swollen joints as well as improving morning stiffness and joint tenderness. A long-term clinical trial found improvements in patient's overall assessment of pain and a reduction in medication, in those patients supplementing with 2.6 g of omega-3 PUFA. Also, patients with rheumatoid arthritis, that were supplemented with 10 g of cod liver oil (containing 2.2 g of omega-3 essential fatty acids) experienced improvements in pain and a reduction in NSAID. The clinical controlled trials do support beneficial effects for supplementing with PUFA, as it can decrease joint inflammation, alleviate morning stiffness, and lower the need for NSAID [17].

Most American diets provide a less than optimal amount of omega-3 PUFA, with a ratio of omega-6 to omega-3 as high as 20:1, as opposed to the 4:1 or 1:1 ratio that is suggested for optimal health. An established mechanism that explains how fish oil has been shown to decrease inflammation is through modifying the class of autacoids (biological factors which act like local hormones) that are produced from fatty acid metabolism through cyclooxygenase (COX) and lipoxygenase

(LOX)-mediated biochemical pathways, from 2-series to 3-series prostaglandins (PG) and 4-series to 5-series of leukotrienes (LT).

Obesity is greatly linked with occurrences of OA in a way that is not proportional to the mechanical overload or abdominal joint stress. There is increasing evidence that adipokine present in individuals suffering from metabolic syndrome and obesity, contribute to the pathobiology of OA. Consumption of fish oil that is rich in omega-3 PUFA has been shown to alter and even improve the adipokine levels and offer chondrocyte and synovial health.

Lopez conducted a clinical trial which looked at individuals with confirmed rheumatoid arthritis or OA of the hip and/or knee, which were consuming 300 mg of krill oil and resulted in reductions of CRP, pain, stiffness, and functional impairment scores based on the Western Ontario and McMaster Universities OA Index. Effects of the krill oil treatment were seen in as few as 7 days and sustained throughout the length of the 30-day study. There are some data that suggest consuming fish oil in a larger dose, to address systemic inflammation and cardiovascular health, in unison with at least 300 mg of krill oil, is an optimal strategy for reducing inflammation and leukocyte infiltration [18].

Bovine chondrocytes reduce cartilage-degrading proteinases (IL-1α, IL-1β and TNF-α), COX-2 and inflammatory cytokines in the presence of n-3 PUFAs, in particular eicosapentaenoic acid (EPA). This helps to provide a molecular explanation that n-3 PUFAs cause a reduction in the mRNA levels for various proteins known to be important in the pathogenesis of OA. Thus, PUFAs may be beneficial in the amelioration of the osteoarthritic symptoms [19].

Animal *in vivo* models have also been used to describe the effects of n-3 PUFA supplementation on OA. Animals that were given a diet rich in n-3 PUFAs for 10-30 weeks, showed a 50% reduction in OA changes. This demonstrates a clear biochemical benefit of n-3 PUFA supplementation in reducing the symptoms of OA which may give further insight into early OA changes in humans [20].

However, the most convincing evidence to support the benefit of n-3 PUFA supplementation for OA is a combination effect of the PUFAs and glucosamine. Those individuals who took 500 mg of glucosamine plus 444 mg of n-3 PUFA experienced 90% less morning stiffness and pain compared to individuals solely taking 500 mg of glucosamine and 444 mg of an oil mixture [21].

Dimethyl Sulfoxide (DMSO)

Dimethyl Sulfoxide (DMSO) is primarily used as an industrial solvent, a manufacturing by-product from the processing of paper. DMSO inhibits the transmission of pain messages through nerves and can be used as a vehicle to help absorb other therapeutic agents through the skin. This particular substance has been used topically for relief from osteoarthritis symptoms, of pain, that functions as an anti-inflammatory agent. One study conducted in Germany applied a 25% gel preparation of DMSO for three weeks daily, which resulted in improvements with pain symptoms during rest and activity, but also revealed side effects of pruritus and skin rash. However, these results have not been replicated in the United States [22].

Although there are favorable data for the use of supplements, the positive effects of nutrients in OA treatment lack higher clinical evidence, with an exception of glucosamine sulfate and chondroitin sulfate.

ROLE OF FUNCTIONAL FOODS FOR PREVENTION AND TREATMENT OF OSTEOARTHRITIS

A functional food is a food or drink product that is consumed as part of the daily diet. It can be separated from traditional food in the idea that it is satisfactorily demonstrated to affect, beneficially, one of more target functions in the body, beyond adequate nutritional effects in a way which is relevant to either the state of well-being and health or the reduction of risks for a disease [6].

A food product can be made into a functional food through one of four ways; eliminating a harmful ingredient, by adding a beneficial ingredient, by increasing the concentration of an ingredient known to have beneficial effects or by increasing the bioavailability or stability of a beneficial ingredient [6].

The American Academy of Nutrition and Dietetics recognizes whole food, plant-based diets as healthy and nutritionally adequate. These diets may provide benefits for preventing and treating certain diseases, such as forms of arthritis.

The plant-based diet shows increased levels of beta and alpha carotenes, lycopenes, lutein, vitamin C, and vitamin E. Ordinary, average diets in the United States incorporate solid and liquid forms of animal proteins; meats and dairy products. Arachidonic acids, found in animal fats, are the precursors to proinflammatory prostaglandins and leukotrienes.

The whole food, plant-based diet is associated with a significant reduction in pain as compared to the traditional American diet or animal and plant foods. Reductions in pain can be seen as early as two weeks after the beginning of the diet modification to solely plant-based foods. A primary mechanism for which the plant-based diet reduces individual-perceived pain can be a result of a normalization of the fatty acid profile and reduced exposure to protein substances that lead to inflammation. In other words, the whole food, plant-based diet drastically reduces the availability of the precursors that produce prostaglandins, thus relieving pain [23].

Soy

Arjmandi and colleges established that soy protein has beneficial effects on OA. Soy protein improved range of motion of the knee joint and symptoms of pain thus showing improvements in quality of life. The pain-reducing properties from the use of soy protein can be attributed to its isoflavones, which are thought to act in a similar manner to estrogen, through estrogen-receptor-mediated events.

Observations of the benefits of soy protein were also observed with milk protein supplementation. Milk supplementation contains milk protein isolates and its effect on OA has yet to be uncovered. However, soy protein still had an effect on cartilage metabolism, which could be due to higher levels of circulating estrogen in women. Estrogen has been shown to suppress synthesis of proteoglycans, which lead to cartilage degradation in OA. However, further investigation on the benefits of soy protein for treatment of OA is still necessary [24].

Studies looking at avocado soy unsaponifiables (ASU) have shown some promising findings for the treatment of OA. Preclinical trials show that, *in vitro*, ASU has an inhibitory effect on IL-1 but stimulation of collagen synthesis in articular chondrocyte cultures. Treatment with ASU can also lead to a reduction in the development of early osteoarthritic cartilage and subchondral bone lesions. The inhibitory effect of ASU on inducible nitric oxide synthase and MMP-13 may be what leads to the reduction in the development of the bone lesions [25 - 27].

Resveratrol and Curcumin

With diseases where inflammation is a primary factor, such as OA, plant derived phytochemicals (*i.e.*, curcumin and resveratrol) have been shown to give therapeutic potential. *Curcumin longa* or turmeric is a plant that is part of the ginger family and a native to Asia. Curcumin (diferuloyl methane) is the most active component in turmeric; containing the anti-inflammatory factor. Turmeric has been used in traditional Indian medicine for many years to treat several diseases including arthritis because of its anti-inflammatory, antioxidant and anti-catabolic effects [28].

Issues of low bioavailability are pronounced when curcumin is given as a drug. In an attempt to increase the bioavailability of curcumin, phosphatidylcholine (found in eggs and soybeans) was paired with curcumin. The pairing was shown to have increased and improved bioavailability and pharmacokinetics, and increased ability to protect the liver as compared with curcumin. Mechanisms behind curcumin's actions involve inhibiting transcription factors such as nuclear factor kappa-light-chain enhancer of activated B cells (NF-kB) and nitric oxide synthase, pro-inflammatory cytokines, and inflammatory factors such as COX-2 and collagenase [28, 29].

Resveratrol, found in the vines, roots, seeds and grape skins, have been shown to possess anti-inflammatory, antioxidant and anti-carcinogenic properties. Resveratrol may have the ability to inhibit the destruction of the joint cartilage; however, it is still difficult to say if a dietary supplement will have the same effects as direct joint injections. Yet, incorporating red grapes and berries can still be beneficial as these types of foods are packed with nutrients and healing properties that can still benefit the individual suffering from OA [30].

A combination of curcumin and resveratrol demonstrated that the pair work best together in suppressing chondrocyte apoptosis and the inhibition of β1-Integrings, which stimulate the mitogen activated protein kinase (MAPK) pathway that is important for chondrocyte survival [31]. These results help to explain the biological mechanisms by which curcumin works to alleviate OA symptoms.

When looking at the effects of curcumin extract on knee pain and function, 180-1500 mg/d of curcumin showed improved scores for pain measured through various pain scales as well as a lower need for NSAIDs [28, 32]. This demonstrates that a higher and lower dosage of curcumin will decrease pain while increasing function of the knee without the negative side effects of taking NSAIDs. Also, curcumin proves to be similarly equal to NSAIDs when individuals were taking either 1500 mg/d of curcumin or 1200 mg/day of ibuprofen as the results on the pain scales showed no difference between the two groups [29]. As individuals experience negative side effects from medications, curcumin may serve as a more tolerable and desirable treatment for those suffering from OA.

CONFLICT OF INTEREST

The authors confirm that the author have no conflict of interest to declare for this publication.

ACKNOWLEDGEMENTS

Declared none.

REFERENCES

[1]   Green J, Hirst-Jones K, Davidson R, *et al.* The potential for dietary -factors to prevent or treat osteoarthritis. Nutrition Society ProcNutr 2014; (73): 278-88.

[2]   Sinusas K. Osteoarthritis: diagnosis and treatment. Am Fam Physician 2012; 85(1): 49-56.
        [PMID: 22230308]

[3]   Gaby AR. Natural treatments for osteoarthritis. Altern Med Rev 1999; 4(5): 330-41.
        [PMID: 10559548]

[4]   Mayo clinic (US). Osteoarthritis. Mayo foundation for medical education and research 2014.

[5]   Miller K, Clegg D. Glucosamine and chondroitin sulfate. Rheumatic Disease Clinics of North America 2011; 37(1): 103-18.
        [http://dx.doi.org/10.1016/j.rdc.2010.11.007]

[6]   Ameye LG, Chee WS. Osteoarthritis and nutrition. From nutraceuticals to functional foods: a systematic review of the scientific evidence. Arthritis Res Ther 2006; 8(4): R127.
        [http://dx.doi.org/10.1186/ar2016] [PMID: 16859534]

[7]   Vista ES, Lau CS. What about supplements for osteoarthritis? A critical and evidenced-based review. Int J Rheum Dis 2011; 14(2): 152-8.
[http://dx.doi.org/10.1111/j.1756-185X.2011.01619.x] [PMID: 21518314]

[8]   Pujalte JM, Llavore EP, Ylescupidez FR. Double-blind clinical evaluation of oral glucosamine sulphate in the basic treatment of osteoarthrosis. Curr Med Res Opin 1980; 7(2): 110-4.
[http://dx.doi.org/10.1185/03007998009112036] [PMID: 7002479]

[9]   Reginster J, Neuprez A, Lecart M, Sarlet N, Bruyere O. Role of glucosamine in the treatment for osteoarthritis. Rheumatol Int Rheumatology International 2012; (32): 2959-67.
[http://dx.doi.org/10.1007/s00296-012-2416-2]

[10]   Henrotin Y, Lambert C. Chondroitin and glucosamine in the management of osteoarthritis: An update. Curr Rheumatol Rep Current Rheumatology Reports 2013; 15(361)

[11]   McAlindon T, Felson DT. Nutrition: risk factors for osteoarthritis. Ann Rheum Dis 1997; 56(7): 397-400.
[http://dx.doi.org/10.1136/ard.56.7.397] [PMID: 9485998]

[12]   Bhattacharya I, Saxena R, Gupta V. Efficacy of vitamin E in knee osteoarthritis management of North Indian geriatric population. Ther Adv Musculoskelet Dis 2012; 4(1): 11-9.
[http://dx.doi.org/10.1177/1759720X11424458] [PMID: 22870491]

[13]   Newnham RE. Essentiality of boron for healthy bones and joints. Environ Health Perspect 1994; 102(7) (Suppl. 7): 83-5.
[http://dx.doi.org/10.1289/ehp.94102s783] [PMID: 7889887]

[14]   Hooshmand S, Arjmandi BH. Viewpoint: dried plum, an emerging functional food that may effectively improve bone health. Ageing Res Rev 2009; 8(2): 122-7.
[http://dx.doi.org/10.1016/j.arr.2009.01.002] [PMID: 19274852]

[15]   Egerbacher M, Wolfesberger B, Gabler C. *In vitro* evidence for effects of magnesium supplementation on quinolone-treated horse and dog chondrocytes. Vet Pathol 2001; 38(2): 143-8.
[http://dx.doi.org/10.1354/vp.38-2-143] [PMID: 11280370]

[16]   Lee CH, Wen ZH, Chang YC, *et al.* Intra-articular magnesium sulfate ($MgSO_4$) reduces experimental osteoarthritis and nociception: association with attenuation of N-methyl-D-aspartate (NMDA) receptor subunit 1 phosphorylation and apoptosis in rat chondrocytes. Osteoarthritis Cartilage 2009; 17(11): 1485-93.
[http://dx.doi.org/10.1016/j.joca.2009.05.006] [PMID: 19490963]

[17]   González-Sarrías A, Larrosa M, García-Conesa MT, Tomás-Barberán FA, Espín JC. Nutraceuticals for older people: facts, fictions and gaps in knowledge. Maturitas 2013; 75(4): 313-34.
[http://dx.doi.org/10.1016/j.maturitas.2013.05.006] [PMID: 23791247]

[18]   Lopez H. Nutritional interventions to prevent and treat osteoarthritis. Part I: Focus on fatty acids and macronutrients. 2012; 4 (5 suppl): 145-54.

[19]   Zainal Z, Longman AJ, Hurst S, *et al.* Relative efficacies of omega-3 polyunsaturated fatty acids in reducing expression of key proteins in a model system for studying osteoarthritis. Osteoarth Cartil 2009; 17(7): 896-905.
[http://dx.doi.org/10.1016/j.joca.2008.12.009] [PMID: 19217322]

[20] Knott L, Avery NC, Hollander AP, Tarlton JF. Regulation of osteoarthritis by omega-3 (n-3) polyunsaturated fatty acids in a naturally occurring model of disease. Osteoarthritis Cartilage 2011; 19(9): 1150-7.
[http://dx.doi.org/10.1016/j.joca.2011.06.005] [PMID: 21723952]

[21] Gruenwald J, Petzold E, Busch R, Petzold HP, Graubaum HJ. Effect of glucosamine sulfate with or without omega-3 fatty acids in patients with osteoarthritis. Adv Ther 2009; 26(9): 858-71.
[http://dx.doi.org/10.1007/s12325-009-0060-3] [PMID: 19756416]

[22] Morelli V, Naquin C, Weaver V. Alternative therapies for traditional disease states: Osteoarthritis. Am Fam Physicians 2003; (67): 339-44.

[23] Clinton CM, OBrien S, Law J, Renier CM, Wendt MR. Whole-foods, plant-based diet alleviates the symptoms of osteoarthritis. Arthritis (Egypt) 2015; 2015: 708152.
[http://dx.doi.org/10.1155/2015/708152] [PMID: 25815212]

[24] Arjmandi BH, Khalil DA, Lucas EA, *et al.* Soy protein may alleviate osteoarthritis symptoms. Phytomedicine 2004; 11(7-8): 567-75.
[http://dx.doi.org/10.1016/j.phymed.2003.11.001] [PMID: 15636169]

[25] Boileau C, Martel-Pelletier J, Caron J, *et al.* Protective effects of total fraction of avocado/soybean unsaponifiables on the structural changes in experimental dog osteoarthritis: inhibition of nitric oxide synthase and matrix metalloproteinase-13. Arthritis Res Ther 2009; 11(2): R41.
[http://dx.doi.org/10.1186/ar2649] [PMID: 19291317]

[26] Appelboom T, Schuermans J, Verbruggen G, Henrotin Y, Reginster JY. Symptoms modifying effect of avocado/soybean unsaponifiables (ASU) in knee osteoarthritis. A double blind, prospective, placebo-controlled study. Scand J Rheumatol 2001; 30(4): 242-7.
[http://dx.doi.org/10.1080/030097401316909602] [PMID: 11578021]

[27] Lequesne M, Maheu E, Cadet C, Dreiser RL. Structural effect of avocado/soybean unsaponifiables on joint space loss in osteoarthritis of the hip. Arthritis Rheum 2002; 47(1): 50-8.
[http://dx.doi.org/10.1002/art1.10239] [PMID: 11932878]

[28] Panahi Y, Rahimnia AR, Sharafi M, Alishiri G, Saburi A, Sahebkar A. Curcuminoid treatment for knee osteoarthritis: a randomized double-blind placebo-controlled trial. Phytother Res 2014; 28(11): 1625-31.
[http://dx.doi.org/10.1002/ptr.5174] [PMID: 24853120]

[29] Kuptniratsaikul V, Dajpratham P, Taechaarpornkul W, *et al.* Efficacy and safety of *Curcuma domestica* extracts compared with ibuprofen in patients with knee osteoarthritis: a multicenter study. Clin Interv Aging 2014; 9(9): 451-8.
[http://dx.doi.org/10.2147/CIA.S58535] [PMID: 24672232]

[30] Mobasheri A, Henrotin Y, Biesalski H, Shakibaei M. Scientific evidence and rationale for the development of curcumin and resveratrol as nutraceuticals for joint health. Int J Mol Sci 2012; (13): 4202-32.

[31] Shakibaei M, Mobasheri A, Buhrmann C. Curcumin synergizes with resveratrol to stimulate the MAPK signaling pathway in human articular chondrocytes *in vitro.* Genes Nutr 2011; 6(2): 171-9.
[http://dx.doi.org/10.1007/s12263-010-0179-5] [PMID: 21484156]

[32]   Nakagawa Y, Mukai S, Yamada S, *et al.* Short-term effects of highly-bioavailable curcumin for treating knee osteoarthritis: a randomized, double-blind, placebo-controlled prospective study. J Orthop Sci 2014; 19(6): 933-9.
[http://dx.doi.org/10.1007/s00776-014-0633-0] [PMID: 25308211]

CHAPTER 4

The Role of Viscosupplementation and Platelet Rich Plasma in the Management of Osteoarthritis of Knee and Hip

Víctor Vaquerizo[1,*] and **Fiona Blanco-Kelly**[2]

[1] *Príncipe de Asturias University Hospital, Alcalá de Henares, Madrid, Spain*

[2] *Fundación Jiménez Díaz University Hospital, Quirón Salud, Madrid, Spain*

Abstract: Osteoarthritis (OA) affects millions of people worldwide. However, there is no consensus on the treatment of OA. Treatments aim to reduce pain and help joint function. But they only improve symptoms in the medium term. Nowadays, we have diverse intra-articular treatments, which aim to get better results. Viscosupplementation and Platelet rich plasma are based on the physiologic relevance of hyaluronic acid in synovial joints, and the effect of platelets in the intra-articular homeostasis respectively. HA is used with good results in young patients with Knee OA grade I-II.

Additionally, there is enough evidence to consider the PRP as a valid and effective treatment to reduce pain and to improve the quality of life of patients with knee OA.

Keywords: Hip osteoarthritis, Hyaluronic acid, Knee osteoarthritis, Platelet rich plasma, Viscosupplementation and growth factors.

INTRODUCTION

The aims of medical treatment of osteoarthritis (OA) are the control of symptoms and to modify the natural history of the disease. Despite different pharmacological treatments that are currently available, they only improve symptoms in the short- and medium term, Hence we have not yet succeeded in modifying OA. All treat-

* **Corresponding author Víctor Vaquerizo:** Príncipe de Asturias University Hospital, Alcalá de Henares, Madrid, Spain; Tel: +34918878121; E-mail: vaquerizovictor@yahoo.es

Ashish Anand (Ed.)

ments have limitations such as the adverse effects of non-steroidal anti-inflammatory drugs (NSAIDs: gastrointestinal, hepatotoxicity and nephrotoxicity) or the loss of efficiency over time.

Nowadays, we have diverse intra-articular treatments; among them, viscosupplementation and Platelet rich plasma, are based on the physiologic relevance of hyaluronic acid in synovial joints and on the effect of platelets in the intra-articular homeostasis respectively.

Action Mechanism of Viscosupplementation

Hyaluronic Acid (HA), also called hyaluronan, is a non-sulfated glycosaminoglycan polysaccharide. HA structure is a polymer chain of disaccharides of different lengths, composed of D-glucuronic acid and D-N-acetylglucosamine [1, 2]. The molecular weight of HA ranges between 5000 and 20 million Da. In the human body the average molecular weight is around 4 million Da. It is soluble in water as a sodium salt. It was discovered in the vitreous humor of bovine eye in 1934.

The HA is part of the connective tissue (which is a major component of the extracellular matrix) and the synovial fluid. It is widely distributed in the human body, being the skin and the cartilage tissues rich in hyaluronic acid, where it plays an important role in the healing processes of wounds and skin injuries [3 - 5].

Synoviocytes are the ones responsible for the synthesis and secretion of HA in the synovial fluid. Between the properties described for HA we can find increasing viscoelasticity, and anti-inflammatory, anabolic, analgesic and chondroprotector effects.

- *Physical Properties*: Hyaluronic acid has viscoelastic properties, which allows the synovial fluid to absorb the impact during movement, whilst it lubricates the joint at rest or in slow movements. However, direct evaluation of kinetics of HA is difficult [5].
- *Anti-inflammatory Effect*: It has an effect on the function of phagocytes, adhesion and stimulation of mitosis. Its administration leads to a decrease of

inflammatory mediators such as Interleukin 1β (IL-1β) and matrix metalloproteinases (MMPs) [6, 7].

- *Analgesic Effect*: An analgesic effect, by inhibiting nociceptors trough substance P, has been observed [3, 8].
- *HA Production*: The application of HA also seems to stimulate the endogenous production of HA by synoviocytes [9, 10]. In OA, a reduction in the concentration and density of HA occurs due to a molecule of smaller size that, causes an alteration in the elastic properties and a decrease, in the synovial fluid, hampering cartilage nutrition.

It is for this reason that a theoretical intra-articular administration would contribute to the restoration of the properties of the synovial fluid, and protect the arthritic joint from further deterioration. In the long term, the reestablishment of joint mobility due to pain relief is thought to trigger a sequence of events, which restores the trans-synovial flow, and subsequently the metabolic and rheological homeostasis of the joint.

There are different commercial compounds such as Hyalgan®, Synvisc®, Durolane®, Euflexxa®. A variety of products have been developed depending on the viscosity and frequency of injections needed [1]. Multiple injections are required, 3 to 5 spaced in 1 to 2 weeks. Although there are new compounds with high-molecular weight HA in a single injection.

The adverse effects (AEs) described in the literature can be classified into local and systemic, and according to literature the rate ranges between 2 and 10% [10, 11]. The most common AEs are local ones, being these erythema, swelling and pain that doesn't exceed more than two days. The greater problem described at this level is the post injection reactive arthritis, typical of the high molecular weight of HA, and characterized by pain, swelling and flushing which appears in the 1.5-7.2% of patients. This reactive arthritis improves with rest, cold and administration of acetaminophen in the first 48-72 hours. In some cases, patients have leukocytosis in the joint fluid, similar to a septic arthritis, although the cultures are sterile. A 1% of cases of septic arthritis have been described. The main systemic adverse effects are hypertension episodes (4%), fatigue (1%), phlebitis and arrhythmias [12].

Action Mechanism of Platelet Rich Plasma

Platelet Rich Plasma (PRP) is defined as "a sample of autologous blood with platelets concentration above baseline values". The first description in the literature was the "Biological glue" described by Matras *et al.* [13] in 1970, where it was described as a biological polymer with fibrinogen, thrombin and calcium. Later on, in 1990 Gibble and Ness [14] introduced the term "Autologous fibrin gel" making emphasis in its haemostatic and adhesive properties. All the tissue cells are in a continuous process of self-renewal. They are embedded in the extracellular matrix, in contact with them, and that actively participates in cellular metabolism and regulation of cell behavior. In this matrix there are morphogenetic proteins and growth factors (GFs), which are responsible for these processes [15].

Platelets are essential in the natural healing process, in inflammatory and cell proliferation phase, and in the subsequent remodeling stage [16], not just for their active participation in haemostasis, but also for its implications in chemotaxis and growth, morphogenesis and cell differentiation. Prior studies have shown that platelets are able to release certain substances that play a vital role in tissue healing and regulating processes like angiogenesis, inflammation and immune response [17]. Platelets contain two types of granules, alpha and dense, with different functions. Once activated, the contents are released by exocytosis through the formation of vesicles in contact with the extracellular matrix. These granules constitute the storage of biologically active proteins [15]. When platelets are activated they secrete the 95% of the presynthesized proteins in an hour. Following this first activation the platelets still release growth factors for a week (Table 1). Platelets contain lysosomes that allow them to synthesize GF and IL. Platelets actively participate in biological functions such as mobilization, adhesion, proliferation, activation and differentiation of mesenchymal cells and other cell types.

As we have mentioned growth factors are polypeptides, which are responsible for regulating mitogenesis, chemotaxis, cell differentiation, and metabolism phenotype of numerous cell types. GFs together with other substances are responsible of activating the healing process. In response to the activation, cells undergo changes in proliferation, differentiation, and protein synthesis with different biological functions [15, 18, 19]. All these processes are defined as "cell activation". Many GFs have been described, transforming growth factor (TGF-β), Insulin-like growth factor-I (IGF-I), platelet-derived growth factor (PDGF), fibroblast growth factor (FGF), vascular endothelial growth factor (VEGF), hepatocyte growth factor (HGF), and tumor necrosis factor-α (TNFα). Growth factors are synthesized by platelets and by other cells. Different studies show how the same GF performs different functions depending on the microenvironment [20]. In fact they can carry opposite actions according to interactions between different growth factors.

Table 1. Cytokines and Proteins present in platelet granules.

Category	Proteins	Biological Function
Adhesive proteins	VWF + pro-peptide, Fibrinogen (Fg), Fibronectin (Fn), Vitronectin (Vn), Thrombospondin-1,-2 (TSP-1, -2), laminin-8	Cell contact interaction, extracellular matrix composition
Proteases and anti-proteases	Tissue inhibitor of metalloprotease 1-4 (TIMPs 1-4), metalloproteinase-1,-2,-4,-9 (MMP-1,-2,-4,-9), ADAMTS13, ADAMS10,17, serpin proteinase inhibitor, platelet inhibitor of FIX, C1 inhibitor, a 1-antitrypsin	Angiogenesis, vascular modelling, regulation of cellular behaviour
Growth and mitogenic factors	Platelet-derived growth factor (PDGF), Transforming growth factor b1and b2 (TGF b1, b2), Epidermal growth factor (EGF), Insulin-like growth factor 1 (IGF-1), Vascular endothelial growth factor A and C (VEGF A, C), Basic fibroblastic growth factor (FGF-2), Hepatocyte growth factor (HGF), Bone morphogenetic protein -2,-4,-6 (BMP-2,-4,-6), CTGF, SCUBE1, IGFBP3	Chemotaxis, cell proliferation and differentiation, angiogenesis

(Table 1) contd.....

Category	Proteins	Biological Function
Chemokines, cytokines and others	RANTES, IL-8, MIP-a, ENA-78, MIP-2, MCP-1, MCP-3, SDF-1a, PF4, b-TG, pro-platelet basic protein (PBP), NAP-2, connective-tissue-activating peptide III T, Angiopoietin-1, High mobility group box 1 (HMGB1), IL-6sR, endostatin, osteonectin, bonesialoprotein, osteoprotegerin	Regulation of angiogenesis, chemotaxis, vascular modelling, cellular interaction, bone formation
Membrane glycoproteins	AlphaIIbbeta 3 (aIIbb3), alphavbeta3 (avb3) PECAM-1, most plasma membrane constituent, receptors for primary agonists, CD63, CD40L, tissue factor, P-selectin, furin, GLUT3, semaphorin 4D, TLT-1, TNF-related apoptosis inducing ligand (TRAIL), syntaxin-2, SANP23	Platelet aggregation and adhesion, endocytosis of proteins, secretion, inflammation, thrombin generation, platelet-leucocyte and platelet-vascular cell interactions
	Dense granules: ATP/ADP, calcium, serotonin, histamine	Fibrin formation, capillary permeability, vascular local regulation

Due to the relationship between growth factors and platelets, we can talk about Plasma Rich in Growth Factors (PRGF). The PRP properties described in the literature include:

- *Haemostasis*
- *Stimulation of Angiogenesis*: Platelets contain pro-angiogenic and anti-angiogenic factors. Have high levels of VEGF, which is one of the most powerful angiogenic factors [21]. But also secrete other factors such as endostatin and PF-4, which are blood vessel formation inhibitors. The works published by different research groups have shown a predominance of the angiogenic effect [22].
- *Cell Proliferation*: They accelerate tissue remodeling. There are chemotaxis factors that act directly on the mobility of stem cells, and promote the migration and activation of these. Among these factors are CD34 +, PDGF, TGF-B. The last one stimulates fibroblast proliferation [23].
- *Anti-Inflammatory*: Different studies show an increase of anti-inflammatory mediators such as lipoxin A4, which inhibits chemotaxis, and migration of

leukocytes. Moreover, the hepatocyte growth factor also has an anti-inflammatory effect through the inhibition of NF-kB's translocation [24].

- *Antimicrobial Potential*: In the alpha granules there are antibacterial proteins known as thrombocidins. They also carry other peptides that are lethal for different bacteria such as *E.coli* or *S. aureus* [25, 26].
- In addition, a recent study demonstrated that PRP increases the HA synthesis by synovial fibroblasts [27].

All PRP preparations have certain steps in common [28]. A specific volume of the patient's peripheral blood, is centrifuged to obtain a concentration of platelets and cytokines over serum baseline. The centrifuged product usually stratifies into 3 layers. The base, named red layer, is filled with erythrocytes; the middle, or buffy coat, contains leukocytes and inflammatory cytokines; the third layer, or yellow layer, represents plasma, platelets, and growth factors [29]. Then the PRP is activated for subsequent injection.

One of the aspects in which there is controversy, is the ideal or minimum platelet concentration to be achieved by PRP. Currently, there are different commercial kits for preparation of PRP. They all have different qualitative and quantitative compositions as showed by their different biological effects (Table **2**), as well as different characteristics based on platelet concentration and presence of leukocytes. There are other differences such as centrifugation, storage and conservation issues. These variables can influence the effectiveness and safety of PRP. In order to standardize the PRP, authors such as Mishra [30] and Delong [31] have proposed two classification systems according to PRP composition.

Table 2. Comparison of different PRP preparation systems.

PRP System (Company)	Formulation	Blood Volume (9ml)	Spin	Time (min)	Platelet increase from Baseline	WBCs	Activator
ACP-OS (Arthrex)	LP-PRP	9	Single	5	x2-3	NO	NO
Fibrinet (Cascade)	LP-PRP	9-18	Single	6	x1-1.5	NO	$CaCl_2$
GPS III (Biomet)	LP-PRP	27-110	Single	15	x2-8	Yes	AT/ $CaCl_2$
PRGF-Endoret (BTI)	LP-PRP	9-54	Single	8	x2-3	NO	$CaCl_2$

(Table 2) contd.....

PRP System (Company)	Formulation	Blood Volume (9ml)	Spin	Time (min)	Platelet increase from Baseline	WBCs	Activator
Regenkit (Regenlab)	LP-PRP	10	Single	9	x1.7	NO	NO/CaCl$_2$
PCCS	LP-PRP		Double		x3-5	Yes	
Vivostat	PRP		Single		x10	NO	NO
Magellan (Medtronic)	LP-PRP	30-60	Double	4-6	x2-5	Yes	CaCl$_2$
SmartPrep (Harvestech)	LP-PRP	20-120	Double	14	x3-4	Yes	BT/ CaCl$_2$

AT: Autologous Trombine, BT: Bovine Trombine

At the present, there are still unresolved questions, such as what should be the optimal concentration of platelets and the centrifugation protocol, or whether leukocytes must include also the activation method. It is recommended that the number of platelets, to obtain the optimal effect, is of between 500,000 and 1,000,000 platelets/µL in PRP. Concentrations below 3.8×10^5 platelets/µL have a suboptimal effect, and concentrations above 1.8×10^6 platelets/µL may have a paradoxically inhibitory effect. Moreover, the presence of leukocytes may have a deleterious effect [32]. The presence of pro-inflammatory ILs as IL-1, IL-8 and IL-9 or metalloproteases (MMP-8 and 9) promote degradation of the extracellular matrix, releasing reactive oxygen free radicals affecting the tissue regeneration. Finally, in relation to the activator, the application of PRP is recommended once activated. The systems usually include CaCl$_2$. Although, the use of bovine thrombin is nowadays contraindicated due to the potential risk of developing coagulopathy, some authors still use it [33].

Clinical Application of HA in Osteoarthritis

Since the beginning of the application of hyaluronic acid in patients with knee osteoarthritis, many studies have tried to show the effectiveness in pain control and the improvement in the quality of life and functional capacity in these patients.

Lately, several reviews have been published. Bellami asserts in his meta-analysis that the application of HA in patients with knee osteoarthritis is safe, with an improvement between the 5th-13th week after the administration [11]. Over the medium term HA has the same effect as NSAIDs and in the long-term the HA has greater benefits when compared with corticosteroids. When we compare the highlights of the different HA by statistical analysis, we observe the heterogeneity of the studied products. First of all, there is a great variability in the degree of chondropathy included; the authors include patients with OA grades I - III, and to our knowledge there is no study that includes patients with grade IV OA according to the Kellgren and Lawrence´s classification (K-L). Additionally, it is difficult to compare the number of infiltrations and the interval between them among the different HA. In the last few years, high-molecular weight HA has been commercialized to reduce the number of injections and therefore the complications. The results achieved with high-molecular weight HA are comparable to those published previously, reducing the complications resulting from the injections.

Different studies show an improvement of 28-54% in the "pain" dimension and of 9-32% for the "functional capacity" dimension of the WOMAC scale. In the study published by Leighton *et al.* [34], the improvement effect of Durolane was over 40% in 50% of the studied patients during the 26 weeks of follow-up. Skwara *et al.* [35] presented an improvement of 23.48% in the Lequesne scale at the 12th week of follow up they used the Ostenil® HA. In 2011, Bannuru [36] argued in his meta-analysis that the HA has a beneficial effect 4 weeks after administration and achieves a maximum effect at the 8th week after treatment, but this effect completely disappears after 24 weeks.

Despite the widespread use of HA, not all studies display good results. Altman *et al.* [37] showed that Durolane presents no statistically significant differences when compared to placebo in the long term. Patients treated with HA showed only significant improvement after 6 weeks. In fact, a stratified analysis showed that only patients with unilateral OA without systemic disease presented a statistically significant response when compared to placebo. Among the recent meta-analysis published, we should mention the review done by Rutjes *et al.* [12] that showed controversial results. They claimed that the use of viscosupplementation has slightly beneficial results; however it presents possible serious adverse effects. After analyzing 89 clinical trials in the last 20 years, only mild clinical improvement in pain with no functional effect was observed in patients with knee OA. They collected a total of 30-50% local complications, and some serious complications such as cardiovascular and gastrointestinal effects. However, they are less than those presented by NSAIDs. The authors wondered about the results of other reviews, evaluating the possibility of the requirements of the clinical trials and the methodology used being the reason for these negative results. The American Academy of Orthopaedic Surgeons (AAOS), in fact, in the Evidence-Based Guideline for the treatment of knee Osteoarthritis [38], does not recommend the use of HA. Although meta-analyses of WOMAC scores found some statistically significant effects, none of the improvements met the minimum thresholds. They report that the most statistically significant difference was observed in high-molecular weight HA.

As a summary of the results achieved in patients with knee OA we can conclude that the HA has positive results in the short and medium term in patients with mild or moderate OA, that the outcome depends on the type of HA, and that it has less complications than NSAIDs.

HA has been in use for more than 25 years, but there are not many studies that cover the use of HA in hip OA. Encouraging, but inconclusive results, have also been observed for the treatment of hip OA. In fact, there is no consensus regarding the molecular weight and density, the number of injections required for long-term results, or the most appropriate indication for injection treatment, concerns which are yet to be clarified. One of the problems regarding treatment is its administration, as this should be performed under real-time ultrasound or fluoroscopic guidance.

Some studies showed an improvement in pain reduction after 3 months of follow-up, which remained until 12 months after treatment. For example, Tikiz et al. [39] observed a reduction in pain of around 40% in the 1st month and clinical improvement during the 6 month follow-up. Migliore et al. [40] showed how the consumption of NSAIDs was reduced in more than 40% and that a statistically significant reduction is maintained up to 24 months when comparing with baseline. The most common side effect was acute local post-injection irritation, whose treatment is addressed by symptomatic measures alone. Secondary granulomatous inflammation has been reported with HA in up to 6% of patients treated with it [41]. Therefore, the use of HA in hip osteoarthritis seems to be safe, well tolerated and has positive results.

Clinical Application of PRP in Osteoarthritis

Over the last 10 years, many studies have been published in the literature, which show the application of PRP in patients with osteoarthritis [42 - 50]. In fact there are several clinical trials comparing the effectiveness of PRP against HA [43, 45, 46, 48, 51, 52]. Despite the results, there are no comparative trials between different kinds of PRP, and therefore it is impossible to assess which PRP system is best. Additionally, there is no consensus on the frequency or the number of injections required.

The first prospective studies [42, 44, 47] showed positive results, with improvements of 30-60% compared to baseline at both 6 and 12 months of follow-up. In fact Filardo *et al.* [44], showed a residual effect up to 24 months of follow up. The best functional results are achieved in young patients and in low cartilage degeneration.

After the preliminary results of early studies, the aim was to assess the effect of platelet-rich plasma compared to the administration of HA [43, 45, 46, 51, 52]. Despite the large number of studies, it is difficult to compare the results as there are some significant differences between them. Some of the problems found are the different types of HA used, the different dosages and the number of injections applied. Moreover, except for some studies that used the same PRP using the technique described by Anitua *et al.*, the PRPs were obtained with different protocols and therefore the number of injections as well as the time between them was different. Finally, if we take into consideration the patients, which were included in the studies, we observe significant differences in age and OA grade, which leads to a very high heterogeneity of patients. There have been many clinical trials carried out in recent years that demonstrate the effectiveness of PRP against HA. According to the results shown by Kon [51], patients treated with PRP showed a statistically significant improvement both at 2 and 6 months of follow-up, being the improvement at 6 months of a 35.6% and a 25.86% in the IKDC scales and EQ-VAS respectively. The percentage of improvement above HA was greater than 10% in both cases. In the study published by Spakova *et al.*

[46] the patients treated with PRP showed an improvement in the WOMAC scale of a 51.36% compared to the 28.48% obtained on the patients treated with HA. In the study by Sánchez [52], which included 176 patients, the patients treated with PRP showed a 35.1% of improvement in the WOMAC scale compared to the 32% in the control group at the end of the 12 months follow-up. Patel *et al.* [53] reported that patients with early bilateral knee osteoarthritis achieved satisfactory results with statistically significant differences between baseline and follow-up scores, in over 64% of patients after 6 months. Patel was the first to compare PRP *versus* placebo. Filardo [49] performed a randomized clinical trial including 109 patients where patients had a significant improvement above the HA after 12 months of follow-up. Cerza [54] analyzed 120 patients including patients with K-L grade 1-3. After 6 months of follow-up patients had an improvement of about 50% when compared to the baseline, and almost 30% when compared to HA. Regarding OA patients with grade III, they showed a significant improvement of about 40% above the HA. Until Vaquerizo´s *et al.* publication, all studies included only patients with low degeneration grades I-II. In fact, Filardo [43, 49] and Kon [44] claimed that the PRP was indicated in young patients with low degeneration.

Vaquerizo *et al.* [55] published a randomized clinical trial including 96 patients. In contrast to previous studies, it included older patients (≥70 years of age) and patients with OA grade IV. It was in the first studies with a follow up of 12 months where patients treated with PRP showed a significant improvement above the 40% compared to HA (Durolane™) at the end of follow-up. Patients with better response were grades 1-2, although patients with OA grade III and IV showed an improvement when compared to HA. Besides, they did not find significant differences between age groups. This study together with other published studies [42, 45, 52], used the same PRP, presenting similar results and therefore an extrapolation of their results could be made. In the study by Raeissadat [56] after a follow-up of 6 months, patients treated with PRP showed an improvement of over a 20% in their quality of life. Moreover, it recognizes that there is a positive response in older patients, although there is a significant inverse relationship between patient´s age and pain reduction. Finally, additional publications (Hart [57] and Say [58]) showed positive results in patients with knee OA treated with PRP when compared to HA and mesocaine treatments, after a 6 months follow-up.

One of the purposes of the OMERAT-OSARSI (Osteoarthritis Research Society International) was to assess the response to treatment in patients with knee OA [59]. They considered as treatment response criteria the reduction of pain or the improvement in function of at least 50%, or absolute changes of more than 20 points on the scale, or an improvement of at least 20% in at least 2 of the following 3 criteria: pain relief, function and overall improvement in scales. Only two studies reference these criteria, Sánchez [52] and Vaquerizo [55]. In Sánchez´s study, 57.3% of the patients responded to treatment. In Vaquerizo´s study, patients treated with PRP presented a significant difference respect HA. The patients of PRGF group improved to 83.33%, of which 54.67% improved at least a 50% in pain or initial functionality.

If we analyze the complications described in the literature, we can observe that PRP has a complications rate of 10-15%, most of them being mild. Authors like Kon [51] or Cerza [54] did not evidence any complications during follow-up, mentioning only pain due to infiltration. Spaková and Patel reported 13.7% patients with pain and stiffness in the knee, which lasted for up to 2 days [46, 53]. Sánchez *et al.* [52] reported a 14.21% of complications. Vaquerizo [55] had an adverse effect rate of 16.67%. The most common complication was pain during infiltration in both groups, a fact that could be due to the injection technique. According Filardo [49], the PRP group presented significantly higher post-injective pain than the HA group. They suggest that this could be due to the presence of leukocytes in the PRP, and therefore proteases; although there is no clear evidence for this.

Despite the good results achieved in recent years and due to the heterogeneity of the PRP analyzed, today different clinical guidelines still exist for the treatment of knee Osteoarthritis [38], as the AAOS guideline, the Evidence-Based Guideline or the latest review [50] which stated that there was insufficient evidence to support the use of platelet-rich plasma injections for patients with knee osteoarthritis in routine clinical practice. In fact, they recommended further clinical trials to provide sufficient evidence.

Only two studies assessing the application of PRP in hip OA have been published. The first one, by Battaglia [60], presents a significant improvement after 3 months when compared to HA in 20 patients, but PRP was not superior at 12 months of follow-up. Recently, Sánchez [61] published another study. After three ultrasound-guided injections of PRP in 40 patients, at the end of the 6 months follow-up, they found a significant reduction in pain levels. A 57.5% of the patients reported a clinically improvement of pain. In fact, 40% of these patients were classified as excellent responders. A 27.5% of the patients did not manifest any benefit after the treatment. Regarding complications, one patient reported a mild rash that disappeared spontaneously and most of the patients reported a transitory feeling of heaviness in the injected joint.

AUTHOR'S OPINION

Nowadays, there is no consensus on the treatment of OA. The scientific evidence questions the use of HA in knee OA. However, this is not so clear in the case of the hip joint. It is still used with good results in young patients with Knee OA grade I-II based on the professional's experience. Nonetheless, in the case of the hip OA, despite the fact that there is no sufficient scientific evidence, infiltration should be considered as an option for patients with pain symptoms who have not yet been listed for joint prosthesis surgery. Further clinical trials are necessary to validate its application in hip OA.

In contrast, although further clinical trials are still recommended, we believe there is enough scientific evidence to consider the PRP as a valid and effective treatment to reduce pain and to improve the quality of life of patients with knee OA. In the case of hip osteoarthritis and due to the small number of studies, there is still not sufficient evidence to support its use, we believe that given such promising initial results it is worth suggesting that further studies should be performed to confirm its utility in hip OA.

CONFLICT OF INTEREST

The authors confirm that the author have no conflict of interest to declare for this publication.

ACKNOWLEDGEMENTS

Declared none.

REFERENCES

[1] Balazs EA, Denlinger JL. Viscosupplementation: a new concept in the treatment of osteoarthritis. J Rheumatol Suppl 1993; 39: 3-9.
[PMID: 8410881]

[2] Alonso Carro G, Villanueva Blaya P. Aplicaciones clínicas y efectos terapéuticos de la viscosuplementación en la artrosis de rodilla. Rev Ortop Traumatol (B Aires) 2002; 5: 458-64.

[3] Waddell DD, Bert JM. The use of hyaluronan after arthroscopic surgery of the knee. Arthroscopy 2010; 26(1): 105-11.
[http://dx.doi.org/10.1016/j.arthro.2009.05.009] [PMID: 20117634]

[4] Punzi L, Schiavon F, Cavasin F, Ramonda R, Gambari PF, Todesco S. The influence of intra-articular hyaluronic acid on PGE2 and cAMP of synovial fluid. Clin Exp Rheumatol 1989; 7(3): 247-50.
[PMID: 2547540]

[5] Gibbs DA, Merrill EW, Smith KA, Balazs EA. Rheology of hyaluronic acid. Biopolymers 1968; 6(6): 777-91.
[http://dx.doi.org/10.1002/bip.1968.360060603] [PMID: 5654612]

[6] Forrester JV, Balazs EA. Inhibition of phagocytosis by high molecular weight hyaluronate. Immunology 1980; 40(3): 435-46.
[PMID: 7429537]

[7] Håkansson L, Hällgren R, Venge P. Regulation of granulocyte function by hyaluronic acid. *In vitro* and *in vivo* effects on phagocytosis, locomotion, and metabolism. J Clin Invest 1980; 66(2): 298-305.
[http://dx.doi.org/10.1172/JCI109857] [PMID: 7400316]

[8] Bagga H, Burkhardt D, Sambrook P, March L. Longterm effects of intraarticular hyaluronan on synovial fluid in osteoarthritis of the knee. J Rheumatol 2006; 33(5): 946-50.
[PMID: 16652425]

[9] Smith MM, Ghosh P. The synthesis of hyaluronic acid by human synovial fibroblasts is influenced by the nature of the hyaluronate in the extracellular environment. Rheumatol Int 1987; 7(3): 113-22.
[http://dx.doi.org/10.1007/BF00270463] [PMID: 3671989]

[10] Reichenbach S, Blank S, Rutjes AW, *et al.* Hylan *versus* hyaluronic acid for osteoarthritis of the knee: a systematic review and meta-analysis. Arthritis Rheum 2007; 57(8): 1410-8.
[http://dx.doi.org/10.1002/art.23103] [PMID: 18050181]

[11] Bellamy N, Campbell J, Robinson V, Gee T, Bourne R, Wells G. Viscosupplementation for the treatment of osteoarthritis of the knee. Cochrane Database Syst Rev 2006; (2): CD005321.
[PMID: 16625635]

[12] Rutjes AW, Jüni P, da Costa BR, Trelle S, Nüesch E, Reichenbach S. Viscosupplementation for osteoarthritis of the knee: a systematic review and meta-analysis. Ann Intern Med 2012; 157(3): 180-91.

[http://dx.doi.org/10.7326/0003-4819-157-3-201208070-00473] [PMID: 22868835]

[13]   Matras H. [Effect of various fibrin preparations on reimplantations in the rat skin]. Osterr Z Stomatol 1970; 67(9): 338-59.
[PMID: 4917644]

[14]   Gibble JW, Ness PM. Fibrin glue: the perfect operative sealant? Transfusion 1990; 30(8): 741-7.
[http://dx.doi.org/10.1046/j.1537-2995.1990.30891020337.x] [PMID: 2219264]

[15]   Alsousou J, Thompson M, Hulley P, Noble A, Willett K. The biology of platelet-rich plasma and its application in trauma and orthopaedic surgery: a review of the literature. J Bone Joint Surg Br 2009; 91(8): 987-96.
[http://dx.doi.org/10.1302/0301-620X.91B8.22546] [PMID: 19651823]

[16]   Anitua E, Andia I, Ardanza B, Nurden P, Nurden AT. Autologous platelets as a source of proteins for healing and tissue regeneration. Thromb Haemost 2004; 91(1): 4-15.
[PMID: 14691563]

[17]   Nurden AT, Nurden P, Sánchez M, Andia I, Anitua E. Platelets and wound healing. Front Biosci 2008; 13: 3532-48.
[PMID: 18508453]

[18]   Reed GL, Fitzgerald ML, Polgár J. Molecular mechanisms of platelet exocytosis: insights into the secrete life of thrombocytes. Blood 2000; 96(10): 3334-42.
[PMID: 11071625]

[19]   Weyrich AS, Prescott SM, Zimmerman GA. Platelets, endothelial cells, inflammatory chemokines, and restenosis: complex signaling in the vascular play book. Circulation 2002; 106(12): 1433-5.
[http://dx.doi.org/10.1161/01.CIR.0000033634.60453.22] [PMID: 12234942]

[20]   Stone DK. Receptors: structure and function. Am J Med 1998; 105(3): 244-50.
[http://dx.doi.org/10.1016/S0002-9343(98)00221-6] [PMID: 9753029]

[21]   Langer HF, Gawaz M. Platelets in regenerative medicine. Basic Res Cardiol 2008; 103(4): 299-307.
[http://dx.doi.org/10.1007/s00395-008-0721-4] [PMID: 18392766]

[22]   Anitua E, Sánchez M, Nurden AT, *et al.* Autologous fibrin matrices: a potential source of biological mediators that modulate tendon cell activities. J Biomed Mater Res A 2006; 77(2): 285-93.
[http://dx.doi.org/10.1002/jbm.a.30585] [PMID: 16400654]

[23]   Anitua E, Troya M, Orive G. Plasma rich in growth factors promote gingival tissue regeneration by stimulating fibroblast proliferation and migration and by blocking transforming growth factor-β--induced myodifferentiation. J Periodontol 2012; 83(8): 1028-37.
[http://dx.doi.org/10.1902/jop.2011.110505] [PMID: 22145805]

[24]   Bendinelli P, Matteucci E, Dogliotti G, *et al.* Molecular basis of anti-inflammatory action of platelet-rich plasma on human chondrocytes: mechanisms of NF-κB inhibition *via* HGF. J Cell Physiol 2010; 225(3): 757-66.
[http://dx.doi.org/10.1002/jcp.22274] [PMID: 20568106]

[25]   Anitua E, Alonso R, Girbau C, Aguirre JJ, Muruzabal F, Orive G. Antibacterial effect of plasma rich in growth factors (PRGF®-Endoret®) against *Staphylococcus aureus* and *Staphylococcus epidermidis* strains. Clin Exp Dermatol 2012; 37(6): 652-7.

[http://dx.doi.org/10.1111/j.1365-2230.2011.04303.x] [PMID: 22329713]

[26] Drago L, Bortolin M, Vassena C, Romanò CL, Taschieri S, Del Fabbro M. Plasma components and platelet activation are essential for the antimicrobial properties of autologous platelet-rich plasma: an *in vitro* study. PLoS One 2014; 9(9): e107813.
[http://dx.doi.org/10.1371/journal.pone.0107813] [PMID: 25232963]

[27] Anitua E, Sánchez M, Nurden AT, *et al.* Platelet-released growth factors enhance the secretion of hyaluronic acid and induce hepatocyte growth factor production by synovial fibroblasts from arthritic patients. Rheumatology (Oxford) 2007; 46(12): 1769-72.
[http://dx.doi.org/10.1093/rheumatology/kem234] [PMID: 17942474]

[28] Wasterlain AS, Braun HJ, Dragoo JL. Contents and formulations of platelet-rich plasma. Oper Tech Orthop 2012; 22(1): 33-42.
[http://dx.doi.org/10.1053/j.oto.2011.11.001]

[29] Anitua E, Andia I, Ardanza B, Nurden P, Nurden AT. Autologous platelets as a source of proteins for healing and tissue regeneration. Thromb Haemost 2004; 91(1): 4-15.
[PMID: 14691563]

[30] Mishra A, Harmon K, Woodall J, Vieira A. Sports medicine applications of platelet rich plasma. Curr Pharm Biotechnol 2012; 13(7): 1185-95.
[http://dx.doi.org/10.2174/138920112800624283] [PMID: 21740373]

[31] DeLong JM, Russell RP, Mazzocca AD. Platelet-rich plasma: the PAW classification system. Arthroscopy 2012; 28(7): 998-1009.
[http://dx.doi.org/10.1016/j.arthro.2012.04.148] [PMID: 22738751]

[32] Weibrich G, Hansen T, Kleis W, Buch R, Hitzler WE. Effect of platelet concentration in platelet-rich plasma on peri-implant bone regeneration. Bone 2004; 34(4): 665-71.
[http://dx.doi.org/10.1016/j.bone.2003.12.010] [PMID: 15050897]

[33] Eming SA, Krieg T, Davidson JM. Inflammation in wound repair: molecular and cellular mechanisms. J Invest Dermatol 2007; 127(3): 514-25.
[http://dx.doi.org/10.1038/sj.jid.5700701] [PMID: 17299434]

[34] Leighton RK, Arden N. A randomized blinded trial comparing one HA injection to corticosteroid for knee osteoarthritis pain. American Academy of Orthopaedic Surgeons, Annual Meeting 2010. PN 640: 583.

[35] Skwara A, Peterlein CD, Tibesku CO, Rosenbaum D, Fuchs-Winkelmann S. Changes of gait patterns and muscle activity after intraarticular treatment of patients with osteoarthritis of the knee: a prospective, randomised, doubleblind study. Knee 2009; 16(6): 466-72.
[http://dx.doi.org/10.1016/j.knee.2009.03.003] [PMID: 19362003]

[36] Bannuru RR, Natov NS, Dasi UR, Schmid CH, McAlindon TE. Therapeutic trajectory following intra-articular hyaluronic acid injection in knee osteoarthritismeta-analysis. Osteoarthritis Cartilage 2011; 19(6): 611-9.
[http://dx.doi.org/10.1016/j.joca.2010.09.014] [PMID: 21443958]

[37] Altman RD, Akermark C, Beaulieu AD, Schnitzer T. Efficacy and safety of a single intra-articular injection of non-animal stabilized hyaluronic acid (NASHA) in patients with osteoarthritis of the knee.

Osteoarthritis Cartilage 2004; 12(8): 642-9.
[http://dx.doi.org/10.1016/j.joca.2004.04.010] [PMID: 15262244]

[38]   Jevsevar DS. Treatment of osteoarthritis of the knee: evidence-based guideline, 2nd edition. J Am
        Acad Orthop Surg 2013; 21(9): 571-6.
        [PMID: 23996988]

[39]   Tikiz C, Unlü Z, Sener A, Efe M, Tüzün C. Comparison of the efficacy of lower and higher molecular
        weight viscosupplementation in the treatment of hip osteoarthritis. Clin Rheumatol 2005; 24(3): 244-
        50.
        [http://dx.doi.org/10.1007/s10067-004-1013-5] [PMID: 15647968]

[40]   Migliore A, Granata M, Tormenta S, *et al.* Hip viscosupplementation under ultra-sound guidance
        riduces NSAID consumption in symptomatic hip osteoarthritis patients in a long follow-up. Data from
        Italian registry. Eur Rev Med Pharmacol Sci 2011; 15(1): 25-34.
        [PMID: 21381497]

[41]   Waddell DD, Beyer A, Thompson TL, *et al.* No conclusive evidence that histologically found
        granulomas and acute local reactions following hylan G-F 20 injections are related or have clinical
        significance. J Knee Surg 2014; 27(2): 99-104.
        [PMID: 23873318]

[42]   Wang-Saegusa A, Cugat R, Ares O, Seijas R, Cuscó X, Garcia-Balletbó M. Infiltration of plasma rich
        in growth factors for osteoarthritis of the knee short-term effects on function and quality of life. Arch
        Orthop Trauma Surg 2011; 131(3): 311-7.
        [http://dx.doi.org/10.1007/s00402-010-1167-3] [PMID: 20714903]

[43]   Kon E, Mandelbaum B, Buda R, *et al.* Platelet-rich plasma intra-articular injection *versus* hyaluronic
        acid viscosupplementation as treatments for cartilage pathology: from early degeneration to
        osteoarthritis. Arthroscopy 2011; 27(11): 1490-501.
        [http://dx.doi.org/10.1016/j.arthro.2011.05.011] [PMID: 21831567]

[44]   Filardo G, Kon E, Buda R, *et al.* Platelet-rich plasma intra-articular knee injections for the treatment of
        degenerative cartilage lesions and osteoarthritis. Knee Surg Sports Traumatol Arthrosc 2011; 19(4):
        528-35.
        [http://dx.doi.org/10.1007/s00167-010-1238-6] [PMID: 20740273]

[45]   Sánchez M, Anitua E, Azofra J, Aguirre JJ, Andia I. Intra-articular injection of an autologous
        preparation rich in growth factors for the treatment of knee OA: a retrospective cohort study. Clin Exp
        Rheumatol 2008; 26(5): 910-3.
        [PMID: 19032827]

[46]   Spaková T, Rosocha J, Lacko M, Harvanová D, Gharaibeh A. Treatment of knee joint osteoarthritis
        with autologous platelet-rich plasma in comparison with hyaluronic acid. Am J Phys Med Rehabil
        2012; 91(5): 411-7.
        [http://dx.doi.org/10.1097/PHM.0b013e3182aab72] [PMID: 22513879]

[47]   Napolitano M, Matera S, Bossio M, *et al.* Autologous platelet gel for tissue regeneration in
        degenerative disorders of the knee. Blood Transfus 2012; 10(1): 72-7.
        [PMID: 22044954]

[48]   Sampson S, Reed M, Silvers H, Meng M, Mandelbaum B. Injection of platelet-rich plasma in patients

with primary and secondary knee osteoarthritis: a pilot study. Am J Phys Med Rehabil 2010; 89(12): 961-9.
[http://dx.doi.org/10.1097/PHM.0b013e3181fc7edf] [PMID: 21403592]

[49]   Filardo G, Kon E, Di Martino A, *et al.* Platelet-rich plasma *vs* hyaluronic acid to treat knee degenerative pathology: study design and preliminary results of a randomized controlled trial. BMC Musculoskelet Disord 2012; 13(1): 229.
[http://dx.doi.org/10.1186/1471-2474-13-229] [PMID: 23176112]

[50]   Laudy AB, Bakker EW, Rekers M, Moen MH. Efficacy of platelet-rich plasma injections in osteoarthritis of the knee: a systematic review and meta-analysis. Br J Sports Med 2015; 49(10): 657-72.
[http://dx.doi.org/10.1136/bjsports-2014-094036] [PMID: 25416198]

[51]   Kon E, Mandelbaum B, Buda R, *et al.* Platelet-rich plasma intra-articular injection *versus* hyaluronic acid viscosupplementation as treatments for cartilage pathology: from early degeneration to osteoarthritis. Arthroscopy 2011; 27(11): 1490-501.
[http://dx.doi.org/10.1016/j.arthro.2011.05.011] [PMID: 21831567]

[52]   Sánchez M, Fiz N, Azofra J, *et al.* A randomized clinical trial evaluating plasma rich in growth factors (PRGF-Endoret) *versus* hyaluronic acid in the short-term treatment of symptomatic knee osteoarthritis. Arthroscopy 2012; 28(8): 1070-8.
[http://dx.doi.org/10.1016/j.arthro.2012.05.011] [PMID: 22840987]

[53]   Patel S, Dhillon MS, Aggarwal S, Marwaha N, Jain A. Treatment with platelet-rich plasma is more effective than placebo for knee osteoarthritis: a prospective, double-blind, randomized trial. Am J Sports Med 2013; 41(2): 356-64.
[http://dx.doi.org/10.1177/0363546512471299] [PMID: 23299850]

[54]   Cerza F, Carnì S, Carcangiu A, *et al.* Comparison between hyaluronic acid and platelet-rich plasma, intra-articular infiltration in the treatment of gonarthrosis. Am J Sports Med 2012; 40(12): 2822-7.
[http://dx.doi.org/10.1177/0363546512461902] [PMID: 23104611]

[55]   Vaquerizo V, Plascencia MÁ, Arribas I, *et al.* Comparison of intra articular injections of plasma rich in growth factors (PRGF-Endoret) *versus* Durolane hyaluronic acid in the treatment of patients with symptomatic osteoarthritis: a randomized controlled trial. Arthroscopy 2013; 29(10): 1635-43.
[http://dx.doi.org/10.1016/j.arthro.2013.07.264] [PMID: 24075613]

[56]   Raeissadat SA, Rayegani SM, Babaee M, *et al.* The effect of platelet-rich plasma on pain, function, and quality of life of patients with knee osteoarthritis. Pain Res Treat 2013; 165967.
[http://dx.doi.org/10.1155/2013/165967]

[57]   Hart R, Safi A, Komzák M, Jajtner P, Puskeiler M, Hartová P. Platelet-rich plasma in patients with tibiofemoral cartilage degeneration. Arch Orthop Trauma Surg 2013; 133(9): 1295-301.
[http://dx.doi.org/10.1007/s00402-013-1782-x] [PMID: 23736793]

[58]   Say F, Gürler D, Yener K, Bülbül M, Malkoc M. Platelet-rich plasma injection is more effective than hyaluronic acid in the treatment of knee osteoarthritis. Acta Chir Orthop Traumatol Cech 2013; 80(4): 278-83.
[PMID: 24119476]

[59]   Pham T, van der Heijde D, Altman RD, *et al.* OMERACT-OARSI initiative: Osteoarthritis Research

Society International set of responder criteria for osteoarthritis clinical trials revisited. Osteoarthritis Cartilage 2004; 12(5): 389-99.
[http://dx.doi.org/10.1016/j.joca.2004.02.001] [PMID: 15094138]

[60]   Battaglia M, Guaraldi F, Vannini F, *et al.* Platelet-rich plasma (PRP) intra-articular ultrasound-guided injections as a possible treatment for hip osteoarthritis: a pilot study. Clin Exp Rheumatol 2011; 29(4): 754.
[PMID: 21906437]

[61]   Sánchez M, Guadilla J, Fiz N, Andia I. Ultrasound-guided platelet-rich plasma injections for the treatment of osteoarthritis of the hip. Rheumatology (Oxford) 2012; 51(1): 144-50.
[http://dx.doi.org/10.1093/rheumatology/ker303] [PMID: 22075062]

CHAPTER 5

Use of Human Amnion/Chorion Allografts in the Treatment of Osteoarthritis

Lauren A. Foy[1], Daniel L. Murphy[2] and Ashish Anand[3,*]

[1] *ATC University of Florida, Florida, USA*

[2] *University of Mississippi Medical Center, Jackson, Mississippi, USA*

[3] *GV Montgomery VA Medical Center, Jackson, Mississippi USA and Assistant Prof(Adj) Department of Orthopedic Surgery, University of Mississippi Medical Center, Jackson, Mississippi, USA*

Abstract: Currently, there is no cure for osteoarthritis (OA). Preliminary treatments focus on symptomatic relief. Initially, patients receive cortisone shots, followed by viscosupplementation in a few weeks. Platelet rich plasma injections are also an option. Surgical options include debridement of joints, osteotomy, arthroscopy, or fusion of the bones. Laboratory studies using rats support the use of amniotic membrane (AM) and chorion membrane (CM) in the regeneration and repair of soft tissues. The potential for CM and AM to moderate osteoarthritis has not been explored in length as yet; however, indirect evidence suggests that they may have advantageous effects on cartilages.

Keywords: Amnion, Arthritis, Chorion, DHACM, Growth factors, Knee, Mesenchymal cells, Placenta, regenerative, Osteoarthritis.

INTRODUCTION

For practitioners treating orthopedic diseases, osteoarthritis (OA) is a frequently encountered pathology. OA is a degenerative joint disease in which the articular cartilage deteriorates, resulting in bone-on-bone contact [1], and it is considered the most common disease of the joints that is associated with high costs [2]. OA

---

* **Corresponding author Ashish Anand:** GV Montgomery VA Medical Center, Jackson, Mississippi USA and Assistant Prof(Adj) Department of Orthopedic Surgery, University of Mississippi Medical Center, Jackson, Mississippi, USA; Tel: 6013624471; Fax: 601 368 4133; E-mail: ashishanandortho@yahoo.com

develops through mineralization of the extracellular matrix (ECM), surface erosion, depletion of proteoglycans (PG), lesion formation, and hypertrophic differentiation of chondrocytes [3]. The loss of articular surface causes joint stiffness and swelling, and as the disease progresses, further sequelae can occur, including bone spur formation around the joint [1]. Ligaments and tendons supporting the joint may also become stiff or weakened secondary to inflammation [1].

Like many disease processes, OA has a pattern of presentation and risk factors. OA has no gender predilection in patients younger than 55 years of age, but is more common in women patients over the age of 55 [1]. There tends to be a familial link, and there is increased prevalence in people who perform repetitive weight-bearing activities [1]. Fractures or trauma to the joint earlier in life can predispose an individual to OA later [1]. Medical conditions that have been associated with OA include hemophilia, which results in bleeding in the joints, decreased or disrupted blood supply to the joints, leading to avascular necrosis, and auto-immune disorders [1].

Symptoms of OA typically begin to manifest during middle age. Almost everyone experiences some degree of symptomatology by age 70 [2]. The most common presenting symptom is pain, especially when the patient is in weight-bearing positions. Patients can sometimes have an audible or palpable grinding and crepitus during specific movement [4]. Stiffness in the morning and after prolonged sedentary activity is common and typically lasts for 30 minutes [4]. This decrease in the range of motion improves upon continued movement; however, over time, there is permanent loss in the degrees of motion. Clinically, the joint can present as swollen and tender, with limited and sometimes severe pain in the range of motion due to bone spurs, pain, or inflammation. A plain radiograph reveals the characteristic "loss of joint space" along with bone wearing or spur formation along the joint line [4].

There is currently no cure for OA [5]. Articular cartilage heals poorly due to its limited capacity for self-repair [6]. Preliminary treatments for OA focus on symptomatic relief. This includes lifestyle changes, such as avoiding repetitive motions, exercising, weight loss, use of assistive devices, and pain management with non-steroidal anti-inflammatory drugs (NSAIDs), pain cream, heat or cold [5]. Physical therapy has the capability to improve range of motion and strengthen supporting joint musculature, but the results vary. Off-loading braces can help by allowing redirection of force transmitted through the joint, decreasing the overall load placed on the joint. However, the off-loading braces can be associated with increased joint damage, pain, and stiffness. Clinical trials have also tested a variety of disease modifying OA drugs (DMOADs), none of which have shown a definitive therapeutic benefit as yet [3]. To find a list of DMOADs currently under clinical trials and their results thus far, the reader is directed to go through the FDA website.

If the conservative methods listed in the previous paragraph fail, injections or surgery are options. Initially, patients receive a series of cortisone shots, followed by viscosupplementation [2]. Platelet rich plasma (PRP) injections are also an option. PRP injections are created by centrifuging the patient's blood and injecting it into the joint space to promote growth factors, cytokines, and adhesive proteins [7]. PRP injections provide additional growth factors, such as transforming growth factor beta (TGF-B1), platelet derived growth factor (PDGF), insulin-like growth factor (IGF), fibroblast growth factor (FGF), epidermal growth factor (EGF), vascular endothelial growth factor (VEGF), and hepatocyte growth factor (HGF) [7]. In addition, PRP injections also contain the cytokine tissue inhibitor of metalloproteinase-4 (TIMP-4), along with the adhesive proteins fibronectin, fibrinogen, vitronectin, thrombospondin-1, and laminin [7]. PRP injections and their therapeutic benefits are discussed in greater detail in a subsequent chapter. Currently accepted surgical options include debridement of the joints *via* arthroscopic surgery, osteotomy to relieve stress on the bone, arthroscopy, or fusion of the bones [1].

In recent years, several studies using rat models support the use of amniotic membranes and chorion in the regeneration and repair of soft tissues. These findings have led to an interest in their use in OA. The potential for chorion and amnion to moderate osteoarthritis has not been explored in length as yet; however, indirect evidence suggests that they may have advantageous effects on cartilage [3]. In this regard, we will discuss two modalities and their therapeutic potential in the treatment of OA: the use of human amniotic membrane cells (HAMCs) and dehydrated human amnion/chorion tissue allografts (dHACM).

PHYSIOLOGY OF THE AMNIOTIC MEMBRANE

The use of amniotic membrane (AM) in the form of HAMCs and dHACM is an appealing therapeutic option for the repair of articular cartilage damage caused by OA. AM is the innermost layer of the amniotic sac, made up of both the amniotic and chorionic membranes [8]. AM has two cellular origins: the amnion epithelial cells (AECs) originate from the embryonic ectoderm, and the amnion mesenchymal cells (MSCs) are derived from the embryonic mesoderm [9]. The amniotic MSCs are isolated and stored for use in regenerating tissues [9]. The terms designated to describe these reservoirs of pluripotent stem cells are the human amnion epithelial cells (HAECs) and human amniotic mesenchymal (HAM) cells. The appeal of using AM is multifactorial. AM is easily accessible and has non-tumorigenic, non-immunogenic, and pluripotent nature [9]. The pluripotent stem cells cultured from AECs have the potential to form the bone, soft tissue, muscle, nerve, fat, or blood vessels [9]. To learn more about the physiology and embryonic origins of AM, specialized text should be referred on the matter.

AMNION EPITHELIAL CELLS AND AMNION MESENCHYMAL CELLS

AECs express molecular markers that suggest their functionality and their origins. For example, AECs express non-polymorphic, non-classical human leukocyte antigen (HLA-G), suggesting similarities with leukocytes, but they lack the polymorphic antigens HLA-A, B, and HLA-DR [9]. They also show markers seen in neuronal, glial cells, and neural progenitors [10]. Amnion and chorion cells express the markers of mesenchymal stem cells, including CD105, CD73, CD90, and fetal-liver kinase, along with CD29, CD166, and very late antigen (VLA)-5 [10]. These markers allude to their mesodermal origins. Amnion and chorion cells also express cell-adhesion markers that are utilized in diapedesis of white blood cells during an inflammatory response. These markers include integrins L-selectin, p-selectin, alpha M beta 2 integrin, CD29, CD44, CD66, VLA-5, and ligand-1 [10]. These common molecular markers suggest that amnion and chorion cells have migration capabilities similar to cells of the immune system [10]. Another unique characteristic of AECs is that they show little allogeneic reactivity. This is due to their lack of CD80 and CD8 expression [9]. AECs can also down-modulate disproportionate inflammation by suppressing T cells, dendritic cells, and B cell function [10]. Finally, AECs are capable of synthesizing and releasing catecholamines and neurotropic factors [10].

Like AECs, MSCs have functionality related to their molecular and structural composition. In particular, MSCs have antimicrobial qualities directly mediated by the secretion of antimicrobial factors LL-37 and indirectly mediated *via* secretion of immunomodulative cytokines [9]. LL-37, also known as cathelicidin, plays a vital role in innate immune defense, specifically against invasive bacterial infections. MSCs also form fibrin and elastin linkages that protect the wounds from infection [9]. The barrier formed by MSCs helps maintain and restore lymphatic integrity, while guarding the circulating phagocytes from exposure, and allows more expedient removal of foreign material from the wound [9]. These properties provide an advantage in surgical wound healing.

AMNIOTIC MEMBRANE USE IN OSTEOARTHRITIS

AM holds considerable promise in a surgical patient. AM decreases scar formation through its effect on fibroblasts, which have an integral role in fibrosis and scar formation [9]. During the process of normal wound healing, neutrophils and macrophages are recruited, which in turn produces cytokines (chemo attractants) that attract fibroblasts [9]. Once fibroblasts have migrated to the site of injury, they are activated by TGF-B1 [9], a chemokine secreted by macrophages and other fibroblasts. TGF-B1 also regulates proliferation, epithelial mesenchymal transition, and immune function, and promotes wound healing [11]. AM down-regulates TGF-B1 and the expression of its receptor by fibroblasts, resulting in decreased fibrosis at the wound [9]. AM also modulates fibroblast activity by secreting VEGF and HGF, which maintains the balance between TGF-1 and TGF-3 in order to help prevent scarring [9]. TGF-1 plays a large role in immune function by inhibiting naïve CD4+ differentiation [9]. The majority of immune cells, specifically leukocytes, secrete TGF-1. TGF-3 is suggested to help regulate cellular adhesion and the formation of the extracellular matrix [9]. In terms of injury, TGF-3 is believed to promote wound healing by the regulation of cellular movement. Overall, these inter-related processes promote tissue reconstruction, rather than scar tissue formation. In addition to its effect on fibroblasts and scar formation, AM has the ability to decrease pain following surgical procedures, by decreasing inflammation and providing a better state of hydration, providing an ideal environment to promote faster healing [9].

HAMCs further modulate the immune response by suppressing the synovial inflammation, improving pain, and decreasing the rate of joint degeneration [12]. The inflammatory response seen with OA is regulated through CD4+ cells, which are implicated in pathologic autoimmune responses. In particular, the Th1 and Th17 subsets of CD4+ cells activate specific pro-inflammatory processes [12]. Th1 cells are the pro-inflammatory effectors of autoimmunity, and Th17 cells are associated with the production of inflammatory mediators [13]. By blunting the effect of these cells, HAMCs decrease inflammation. HAMCs also stimulate the generation of CD4+, CD25+, and FoxP3+ T-reg cells, which have the ability to suppress collagen-specific T-cell responses [12]. In summary, systemic infusion of HAMCs significantly decreases the occurrence as well as the severity of collagen-induced arthritis by down-regulating Th1 driven autoimmunity and inflammation [12]. HAMCs also decrease the production of a variety of inflammatory cytokines and chemokines in the joints, impaired antigen-specific Th1/Th17 cell expansion within the lymph nodes, and peripheral antigen-specific T-reg cells [12].

In addition to the inflammatory properties, AM has the potential to be used in the treatment of OA through cartilage repair. When the articular cartilage is injured, even though it has limited capacity for self-healing, cryo-preserved HAMCs can be beneficial in cartilage tissue repair [6]. Cryo-preserved HAMCs bond well with native cartilages and provide a more regular surface to function as a scaffold for growing human chondrocytes [6]. This helps facilitate repair of the cartilage.

DHACMS CHEMICAL COMPOSITION

dHACMs are the biologically active dehydrated human allograft comprised of laminated amnion and chorion membranes [14]. These allografts retain soluble biological molecules that promote dermal fibroblast and microvascular endothelial cell proliferation, chemotactic recruitment of MSCs, and up-regulation of angiogenic growth factors by endothelial cells, thereby promoting healing [8]. dHACMs contain factors capable of stimulating naïve MSC migration and recruitment [15]. In addition, dHACMs contain at least three tissue inhibitors of metalloproteinase (TIMPs), which directly inhibit matrix metalloproteinase (MMP) activity. MMPs play a major role in tissue remodeling and degradation of ECM components [15]. They are atypically elevated in many chronic wounds [15]. Inhibiting MMPs minimizes ECM degradation, allowing faster wound healing and less scar formation [15]. In summary, some of the efficacy of dHACMs in wound healing is due to the presence of TIMPs *via* the inhibition of MMPs activity, causing a shift from degradation to synthesis, and therefore restoration of an extracellular matrix [15]. This multifaceted tissue graft affects multiple physiological processes, including but not limited to inflammation, cell proliferation, metalloproteinase activity, and recruitment of stem cells [15].

An enzyme-linked immunosorbent assay (ELISA) performed on the dHACMs shows quantifiable levels of a number of pro-angiogenic growth factors [15]. These growth factors include: angiogenin, angiopoietin 2 (ANG-2), EGF, basic fibroblastic growth factors (bFGF), heparin binding epidermal growth factor (HB-EGF), HGF, platelet derived growth factor BB (PDGF-BB), placental growth factor (PIGF), VEGF, and interleukins (IL-4, -6, -8, and -10) [14]. EGF promotes angiogenesis and induces epithelial development [11]. TGF-a stimulates cell division for fibroblasts, induces epithelial development, and is a more potent angiogenic factor and a stimulator for keratinocyte migration [11]. TGF-B1, as mentioned previously in the chapter, is suggested to regulate proliferation and epithelial mesenchymal transition, and promotes immune function along with wound healing [11]. bFGF promotes proliferation and angiogenesis and induces cell growth and migration, along with assisting in pattern formation, and aids in metabolic regulation, neurotrophic effects, and tissue repair [11]. PDGF primarily promotes cell division and wound healing [11]. VEGF induces angiogenesis and increases micro-vascular permeability [11]. Although the ELISA results show an array of growth factors, in order for the growth factors in the dHACMs to be distributed to the wound, they must enter the wound either by simple diffusion or by tissue remodeling. As mentioned before, dHACM implants are associated with progenitor cell migration to the implant site, which helps transport the growth factors from the allograft to the wound bed.

COLLECTION OF TISSUE

The placentas used for the allograft collection are donated following routine cesarean sections after informed consent [14]. Donation is in accordance with the Food and Drug Administration's (FDA) Good Tissue Practice, along with the American Association of Tissue Banks (AATB) [14]. In order to qualify for donation, all donors have to test negative for infectious disease: hepatitis B and C, syphilis, cytomegalovirus (CMV), human immunodeficiency virus (HIV), and human T-lymphotropic virus (HTLV) [14]. After testing negative, the amnion and chorion are isolated from the placenta. Most tissues are sterilized using the Purion© process [11]. This specific dehydration process allows the tissue to retain the natural growth factors and regulatory molecules of the amnion and chorion [11]. After cleansing, the membrane layers are laminated to form the graft [8]. This graft is then dehydrated under controlled drying conditions [8]. This meticulous process preserves the elements associated with increased wound healing. For greater detail about the collection process, please refer to product specific texts.

Once dehydrated, the dHACMs can be stored at room temperature for up to five years in the form of a sheet or be micronized to create a powder form [14]. One benefit of the sheet is its flexibility, which allows it to conform to irregular surfaces [16]. The sheet can also be sutured, taped, stapled, or glued, depending on surgeon preference [16]. A micronized form of dHACMs was also recently developed. When ready to be used, this can be mixed into a topical powder or combined with normal saline and injected into the joint space.

Micronized dHACMs have been shown to contain all same growth factors as in the sheet form [16]. Micro-CT imaging after the use of micronized dHACMs in rodents showed significant decreases in cartilage destruction *via* higher proteoglycans levels, a smaller quantity of erosions, and no lesions [3].

LIMITATIONS

The limitations of using the sheet form of dHACMs made research difficult and resulted in a paucity of previous investigative studies in OA [3]. Sheets are used to treat large defects and required invasive surgery, which is difficult to perform on rats [3]. Since the creation of micronized dHACMs, research has become less challenging, due to the minimally invasive administration technique.

Another challenge when considering the use of DMOADs is particle size. If the particles are too small, they distribute to spaces outside the joint through the intracellular gaps or are phagocytized by macrophages [3]. If the particles are too large, they have the potential to initiate immune response or cause damage to the articular surface [3]. Currently, research is trying to prevent rapid clearance of micronized dHACMs by adding biomaterials to the solution. These biomaterials include poly-lactic glycolic acid, albumin, and biopolymer-based carriers [3].

dHACMs are not a perfect solution to the problem of osteoarthritis. Patients may lack healthy chondrocytes, precluding regeneration. In addition, the implantation technique may cause additional damage to the joints [6]. In addition, the mechanism for chronic wound formation is poorly understood at the molecular level. Inflammation, angiogenesis, and cell-mediated regeneration of vasculature are complex and interrelated physiological processes that require a well-coordinated sequence of events to promote healing. The over-lapping functions and complexity of the growth factors present in HAM make assignment of biological activity to specific molecules impossible. In this sense, using amniotic membranes is like using a coarse approach to a finely tuned process.

CONCLUSION

The physiologic benefits of using dHACMs are the anti-microbial, anti-angiogenic, anti-inflammatory, and anti-tumor properties, which reduce pain and improve scarring. In addition, the amnions of HAM contain many of the components of natural cartilage, promoting healing. Moreover, HAM has no immune response, reducing the risk of rejection associated with transplantation. When compared to the platelet-rich plasma injections, HAM contain cytokines, elastin, and collagen, which promote better wound healing. The combination of growth factors found in dHACM have also been shown to act synergistically to further enhance the wound healing response, so it is more effective in achieving the biological coordination required for accelerated wound healing. The efficacy of dHACMs contributes to their proven cost effectiveness when compared to growth factor treatments alone. HAM has sparked great interest over recent years, particularly in regenerative medicine. To learn more about specific products and costs please refer to the specific dHACM producers' manuals.

CONFLICT OF INTEREST

Lauren Foy and Daniel Murphy confirm that this chapter contents have no conflict of interest. Ashish Anand confirms that he has made paid presentations for Mimedx as member of Speakers Bureau-but none pertaining to the content of the chapter. None of the above authors have stock options.

ACKNOWLEDGEMENTS

Declared none.

REFERENCES

[1]   Lane NE, Schnitzer TJ. Osteoarthritis. In: Goldman L, Schafer AI, Eds. Goldman's Cecil Medicine. 24th ed., Philadelphia, Pa: Elsevier Saunders 2011.

[2]   Bijlsma JW, Berenbaum F, Lafeber FP. Osteoarthritis: an update with relevance for clinical practice. Lancet 2011; 377(9783): 2115-26.
[http://dx.doi.org/10.1016/S0140-6736(11)60243-2] [PMID: 21684382]

[3]   Willett NJ, Thote T, Lin AS, *et al.* Intra-articular injection of micronized dehydrated human amnion/chorion membrane attenuates osteoarthritis development. Arthritis Research & Therapy 2014; 16(1): R47.

[4]   Nelson AE, Jordan JM. Clinical features of osteoarthritis. In: Firestein GS, Budd RC, Gabriel SE, Eds. Kelly's Textbook of Rheumotology. 9th ed., Philadelphia, Pa: Elsevier Saunders 2012.

[5]   Hochberg MC, Altman RD, April KT, *et al.* American College of Rheumatology 2012 recommendations for the use of nonpharmacologic and pharmacologic therapies in osteoarthritis of the hand, hip, and knee. Arthritis Care Res (Hoboken) 2012; 64(4): 465-74.
[http://dx.doi.org/10.1002/acr.21596] [PMID: 22563589]

[6]   Díaz-Prado S, Rendal-Vázquez ME, Muiños-López E, *et al.* Potential use of the human amniotic membrane as a scaffold in human articular cartilage repair. Cell Tissue Bank 2010; 11(2): 183-95.
[http://dx.doi.org/10.1007/s10561-009-9144-1] [PMID: 20386989]

[7]   Sanchez-Gonzalex DJ, Mendez-Bolaina E. Tejo-bahena. Platelet-rich plasma peptides: Key for

regeneration. Int J Pept 2012; 2012: 532519.

[8]   Koob TJ, Lim JJ, Massee M, Zabek N, Denoziere G. Properties of dehydrated human amnion/chorion composite grafts: Implications for wound repair and soft tissue regeneration. J Biomed Mater Res Part B 2014; 102(6): 1353-62.

[9]   Chopra A, Thomas BS. Amniotic membrane: A novel material for regeneration and repair. J. Biomim. Biomater. Tissue Eng. 18: 106. doI:10:4172/1662-100x 1000106

[10]   Bailo M, Soncini M, Vertua E, *et al.* Engraftment potential of human amnion and chorion cells derived from term placenta. Transplantation 2004; 78(10): 1439-48.
        [http://dx.doi.org/10.1097/01.TP.0000144606.84234.49] [PMID: 15599307]

[11]   AmnioFix (US). Scientific & Clinical Compendium 2013.

[12]   Parolini O, Souza-Moreira L, OValle F, *et al.* Therapeutic effect of human amniotic membrane-derived cells on experimental arthritis and other inflammatory disorders. Arthritis Rheumatol 2014; 66(2): 327-39.
        [http://dx.doi.org/10.1002/art.38206] [PMID: 24504805]

[13]   Damsker JM, Hansen AM, Caspi RR. Th1 and Th17 cells: adversaries and collaborators. Ann N Y Acad Sci 2010; 1183: 211-21.
        [http://dx.doi.org/10.1111/j.1749-6632.2009.05133.x] [PMID: 20146717]

[14]   Koob TJ, Lim JJ, Massee M, *et al.* Angiogenic properties of dehydrated human amnion/chorion allografts: therapeutic potential for soft tissue repair and regeneration. Vasc Cell 2014; 6: 10.
        [http://dx.doi.org/10.1186/2045-824X-6-10] [PMID: 24817999]

[15]   Koob TJ, Rennert R, Zabek N, *et al.* Biological properties of dehydrated human amnion/chorion composite graft: implications for chronic wound healing. Int Wound J 2013; 10(5): 493-500.
        [http://dx.doi.org/10.1111/iwj.12140] [PMID: 23902526]

[16]   Alliqua Biomedical (US). Tissue Reborn: Brining the regenerative power of the amnion to tissue restoration 2014.

CHAPTER 6

Role of Cartilage Regeneration in the Management of Early Knee Arthritis: Current Concepts

Mark F. Sommerfeldt, Avijit Sharma and **David C. Flanigan**[*]

OSU Sports Medicine and Cartilage Restoration Program, The Ohio State University Wexner Medical Center, Columbus, Ohio, USA

Abstract: In this chapter, we discuss review cartilage restoration surgery in the setting of early knee osteoarthritis (OA). We introduce an algorithmic approach to determining treatment and discuss procedures including microfracture, autologous matrix-induced chondrogenesis (AMIC®), osteochondral autograft transfer (OATS), osteochondral allografting (OCA), autologous chondrocyte implantation (ACI)/matrix-assisted chondrocyte implantation (MACI), and stem cell therapy. These techniques have particular advantages and disadvantages. The authors share their approach and outline the protocol for postoperative rehabilitation.

Keywords: ACI, AMIC, Cartilage, MACI, Microfracture, OATS, OCA, Osteoarthritis, Rehabilitation, Stem cell therapy.

INTRODUCTION

Osteoarthritis (OA) is a degenerative joint disease characterized by the breakdown and ultimate loss of articular cartilage [1, 2]. It is extremely common, with an estimated prevalence of 27 million in the United States [3]. The knee is commonly involved, and symptoms of knee osteoarthritis include pain and swelling and often lead to functional loss and disability [4]. One of the pathways to OA includes focal cartilage breakdown or defect [5]. Focal defects have been found in 7% of patients under the age of 40 at the time of arthroscopy and 9% of patients under

[*] **Corresponding author David C. Flanigan:** OSU Sports Medicine and Cartilage Restoration Program, Department of Orthopaedics, The Ohio State University Wexner Medical Center, Columbus, Ohio, USA; Tel: (614) 293-2412; Fax: (614) 293-4755; E-mail: david.flanigan@osumc.edu

Ashish Anand (Ed.)

the age of 50 [6]. Often these cartilage defects are associated with other pathology, including meniscus tears and knee instability [6].

The initial management of early knee OA includes weight loss, activity modification, physical therapy, bracing, oral analgesics, and intra-articular injections (corticosteroid or hyaluronic acid). These treatments are designed to decrease symptoms and delay total knee arthroplasty (TKA) until a point is reached at which the benefit of such a procedure outweighs the risk [4, 7].

In recent years, much attention has been paid to joint-preserving techniques. If one could reverse or slow early arthritic cartilage loss, tremendous benefit could be provided to many people living with early OA. The purpose of this chapter is to review cartilage restoration surgery in the setting of early knee OA.

An algorithmic approach will be presented followed by a brief discussion about the following cartilage restoration procedures: microfracture, autologous matrix-induced chondrogenesis (AMIC®), osteochondral autograft transfer (OATS), osteochondral allografting (OCA), autologous chondrocyte implantation (ACI)/matrix-assisted chondrocyte implantation (MACI), and stem cell therapy. Techniques will be described along with advantages and disadvantages of each. The authors approach will be outlined along with their postoperative rehabilitation protocol.

ALGORITIIM

In many ways, the approach to focal early osteoarthritic cartilage defects is similar to the algorithmic approach to traumatic cartilage defects (Fig. **1**) [8]. This algorithm is contingent on both patient-specific and lesion-specific factors in deciding between palliative, reparative, and restorative approaches [8 - 12]. Patient age, expectations, and activity level significantly influence treatment decisions. Patient sex and body mass index (BMI) are other factors that may influence outcomes [12].

Younger patients are likely to have better results after cartilage restoration surgery than older patients, especially after microfracture [13, 14]. Defect size, defect location, involvement of the subchondral bone, and presence of an intact peripheral rim *versus* diffuse changes are lesion-specific factors that the surgeon needs to assess before offering cartilage surgery to any patient.

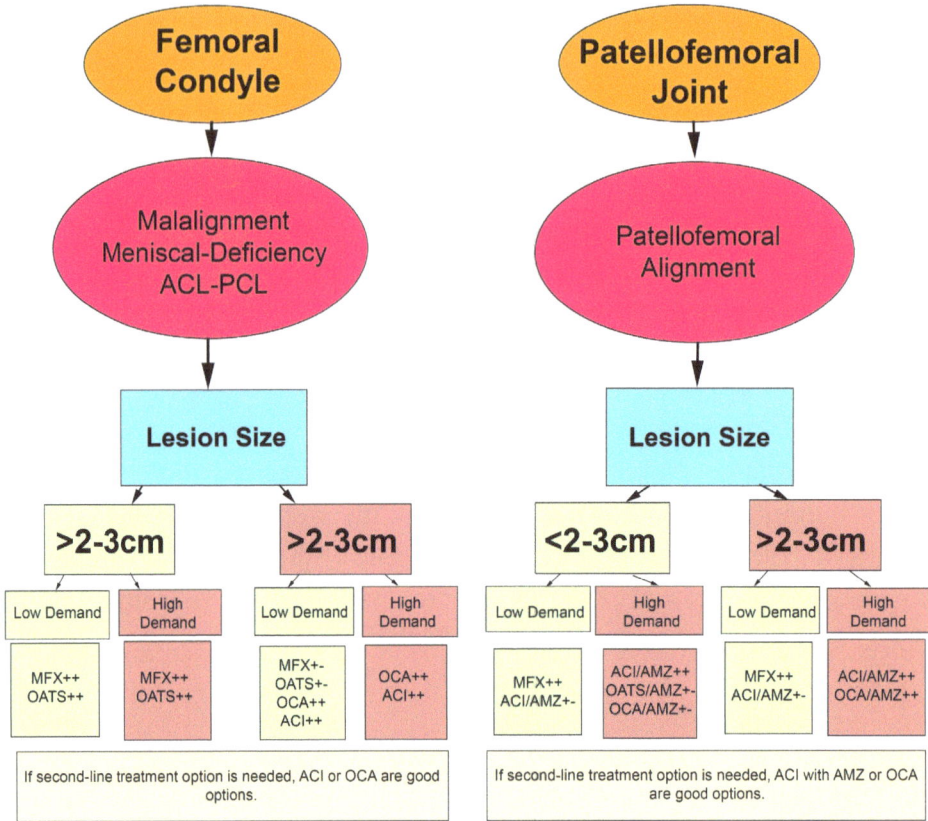

Fig. (1). Treatment algorithm for focal chondral lesions. Before treatment, it is important to assess the presence of correctable lesions. Surgical treatment should be considered for trochlear and patellar lesions only after use of rehabilitation programs has failed. The treatment decision is guided by the size and location of the defect, the patient's demands, and whether it is first- or second-line treatment. ACL = anterior cruciate ligament, PCL = posterior cruciate ligament, MFX = microfracture, OATS = osteochondral autograft transplantation, ACI = autologous chondrocyte implantation, OCA = osteochondral allograft, AMZ = anteromedialization, ++ = best treatment option, and +− = possible option depending on patient's characteristics. Reprinted with permission from Cole BJ, Pascual-Garrido C, Grumet RC. Surgical management of articular cartilage defects in the knee. J Bone Joint Surg Am. 2009 Jul;91(7):1778-90.

Isolated factors, such as patient age, should be considered but should not arbitrarily influence treatment decisions. For example, one could argue that a well-motivated, healthy 58-year-old individual with an isolated, focal chondral defect and an otherwise normal knee should still be a surgical candidate, despite being at an age at which many insurance companies are hesitant to fund his surgery. On the other hand, a 48-year-old sedentary patient with end-stage tri-compartmental osteoarthritis is not likely to be an ideal candidate for cartilage restoration surgery with current techniques.

All of these factors are assessed when determining what the best treatment choice is for the patient given his goals and expectations. It is important to understand that multiple techniques can be indicated for a patient, but determining the best choice may be dependent upon initial diagnostic arthroscopy. Patients should be advised that complete recovery can take more than 24 months and that compliance with postoperative rehabilitation is essential to success. Co-existing pathology such as ligamentous instability, meniscus deficiency, and malalignment need to be considered and in many cases addressed in conjunction with cartilage surgery for best results. In general, the main techniques used for cartilage regeneration include: marrow-stimulating techniques (microfracture, AMIC®), osteochondral autograft, autologous chondrocyte implantation (ACI/MACI), and osteochondral allografts.

MICROFRACTURE

Microfracture is a commonly employed marrow stimulation technique that was initially described by Steadman [15, 16]. By creating bleeding holes in the base of a cartilage defect, a clot can form and pluripotent cells from the marrow space can migrate to fill the defect with a fibrocartilagenous repair tissue [17].

The technique involves arthroscopically debriding loose cartilage with a shaver and a curette to create a stable rim which is required to contain the subsequent clot. The calcified cartilage layer is then removed with a curette; a burr may be needed to remove sclerotic bone until punctate bleeding is achieved. An awl is then used to make holes 3-4 mm apart and 2-4 mm deep. Adequate hole depth is confirmed by the emergence of marrow fat droplets from the holes [15, 18].

Many reports show that when used for traumatic chondral defects, microfracture can reliably lead to clinical improvements in the short-term that tend to decline with time [16, 19 - 22]. Microfracture has also been investigated for use in early OA defects. These published reports generally show improvements in clinical scores from baseline levels over the short term that decline in the long term [23 - 26]. Two factors that were found to relate to the rate of survival were size of the defect and amount of preoperative varus malalignment [26].

The limited durability of microfracture is attributable to the quality of repair tissue formed in the osteoarthritis defect [27, 28]. Kaul *et al.* and Sakata *et al.* performed histochemical analysis of tissue from osteoarthritic lesions after failed microfracture surgery at the time of TKA. Repair tissue was found to be primarily fibrocartilagenous with significant differences from normal hyaline cartilage.

Microfracture has also been used in conjunction with other techniques for the treatment of early osteoarthritic cartilage defects. Combining medial opening wedge high-tibial osteotomy (HTO) with microfracture for the treatment of varus medial compartment OA has been shown to be an effective means of improving clinical outcomes and delaying TKA in some studies [29, 30], although one study suggests HTO alone yields similar results [31]. Sterett *et al.* found that survivorship, as defined by not needing TKA, was 97% at 5 years, and 91% at 7 years after HTO and microfracture. Alteration of the joint reaction forces through the medial compartment by shifting the mechanical axis is the likely explanation. Lee *et al.* performed a randomized controlled study comparing microfracture to microfracture plus platelet-rich plasma (PRP) injection for early OA in 49 patients over the age of 40 with lesions less than 4 cm^2 [32]. Both groups improved significantly, but more knees were rated as normal in the experimental group. The authors concluded that PRP provides growth factors in a one-step, cost-effective way.

The advantages of microfracture include its simplicity, its cost-effectiveness, and its demonstrated safety profile. It is an entirely arthroscopic one-stage procedure that avoids donor site morbidity. The disadvantages of microfracture include its limited durability, which stems from its inability to re-reproduce hyaline cartilage, and its poor results with large lesions.

AMIC®

AMIC® is a novel technique that is thought to enhance microfracture by using a membrane that protects the clot and acts as a matrix for cartilage formation [33 - 36]. The focal cartilage defect needs to be prepared in a manner similar to microfracture. Following microfracture, a collagen I/III membrane (Chondro-Gide®, Geistlich Pharma AG, Switzerland) is sewn onto the defect, which contains the clot and cells and acts as a scaffold. It was originally described as an alternative to ACI when ACI was unavailable due to cost or other reasons [36, 37].

Short- and mid-term results of AMIC® procedures for focal cartilage defects have been published and generally show improvements in clinical scores from pre-operative levels to most recent follow-up in most patients [33, 34]. A randomized control trial that compared AMIC® to microfracture found that the two techniques yielded similar results over the short term; however, long-term studies are required before conclusions about AMIC® can be made [38]. No reported studies have reported on the results of AMIC® for strictly early OA cartilage defects. Of the reported case series, Gille *et al.* included the oldest patients (up to age 61) [33]. Despite holding promise, the use of AMIC® in the management of early OA remains experimental.

One advantage of the procedure is its ability to be completed in a single stage. Relative to ACI, it is much less costly. Its most limiting disadvantage is lack of long-term results.

OATS

OATS is a technique that involves the transfer of an osteochondral plug or plugs from a non-weightbearing portion of the knee to the site of a cartilage defect. It originated in the late 1990s as a one-step operation for the treatment of cartilage defects of the weight-bearing surfaces of the knee [39, 40]. When multiple plugs are used to fill a large defect, it is called mosaicplasty.

The procedure begins by debriding the edges of a cartilage defect to healthy margins. A tubular chisel is used to create a round hole at the site of the defect. A properly sized chisel is then similarly tapped into the donor site, which is usually either the medial border of the medial condyle or lateral border of the lateral condyle. Care must be taken to ensure appropriate width and depth of the donor plugs. A guide is then used to deliver the graft into a slightly dilated recipient tunnel, and a plunger is used to match the surface of the graft to the surrounding cartilage [41].

Initial reports for mosaicplasty for traumatic osteochondral defects were quite promising with good-to-excellent results reported in between 79-92% of patients [41]. A randomized control trial of OATS and microfracture in athletes under the age of 40 found significantly better results and a higher return to play rate in the OATS group [13, 42]. The first study that compared mosaicplasty to ACI found that results after mosaicplasty deteriorated significantly over time, compared to ACI [43]. The authors concluded that OATS should not be used in patellofemoral defects, because of poor results for these defects, and that it might be best used for small (<1cm^2) defects. Other studies, however, have found that OATS is comparable to ACI for defects of various sizes [44, 45]. A case series that investigated OATS for osteoarthritic defects found good results in patients with a solitary OA defect but poor results in patients with multi-focal OA [46].

Advantages of OATS are that it is completed in a single stage and that it restores normal hyaline cartilage to the site of the defect. Additionally, it is able to restore the normal osteochondral tidemark. Disadvantages include donor site morbidity, fibrocartilage formation at the edges of the graft, and the potential for graft incongruity or cartilage thickness mismatch.

OCA

OCA has been used for decades for multiple reasons, including osteochondral defects secondary to trauma, tumor and OA [47, 48]. Typically, OCA is used for lesions larger than 2 cm^2 [8]. Modern OCA is in many ways similar to OATS, except that the donor plug is harvested from a matching location on an allograft specimen. Shell grafts are indicated when defects are inaccessible (such as on the posterior femoral condyles), and involve shaping the graft and securing them with rigid fixation [49]. Issues pertaining to graft procurement, processing and storage do add complexity and cost. Due to concern about decreasing chondrocyte viability with prolonged storage, the process of obtaining the graft and implanting it is time sensitive [49]. Most grafts used today are fresh or fresh frozen, and efforts are being made to optimize their chondrocyte viability, as well as their shelf-life [49]. In young patients with post-traumatic defects of the femoral condyles, OCA has shown encouraging results with a reported survivorship of 95%, 85%, and 74% after 5, 10, and 15 years, respectively [50]. Unfortunately, results have not been as promising for OA cartilage lesions and success rates have been reported to be 30-42% [51, 52]. This highlights the limitation of using OCA for focal cartilage lesions rather than a diffusely arthritic knee. Evaluation of preoperative radiographs and arthroscopic findings can be used to determine if a patient is well suited for OCA.

Advantages and disadvantages of OCA are in many ways the same as those for OATS. Additionally, the donor site morbidity of OATS is avoided while maintaining versatility in terms of plug sizes. Additional disadvantages include the risk of disease transmission, cost, availability, limited chondrocyte viability, and limited documented success in the setting of OA.

ACI/MACI

Autologous chondrocyte implantation (ACI) was first introduced in Sweden in the late 1980s [53, 54]. It was devised for the purpose of restoring articular cartilage into a cartilage defect.

To perform the technique, chondrocytes are first harvested from a healthy part of the knee during arthroscopy. These cells are isolated and cultured for 14-21 days before being prepared for re-implantation. At a second surgery, the defect is prepared by excising all damaged cartilage and using a scalpel to make a vertical rim of healthy cartilage. A ring curette is then used to debride the calcified cartilage layer. With the defect prepared, a template is then used to measure its size. In first generation ACI, a periosteal flap is then harvested from the proximal medial tibia and sutured over the defect. The autologous chondrocytes are then injected under the flap, which must be secured with a water-tight closure. The second generation of ACI utilizes a collagen I/III patch (Chondro-Gide®, Geistlich

Pharma AG, Switzerland), rather than a periosteal flap and has been found to have a lower rate of graft hypertrophy [55]. The third generation of ACI is referred to as MACI, and involves seeding the cells onto a scaffold matrix prior to implantation, which negates the need for suturing and allows for an all-arthroscopic technique [56].

Initial results of ACI in young patients were quite promising [54]. Good-to-excellent clinical results were seen in 65-92% of patients, with the best results seen in patients with femoral condylar defects. Arthroscopic findings suggested good tissue fill, integration, and hardness. Hyaline-like tissue was identified on histologic analysis in most cases [54]. At long-term follow-up, similarly encouraging results have been reported, with 92% of patients satisfied and willing to have ACI again [57]. There remains a need for long-term controlled studies to confirm these results. Critical to the success of this procedure is patient selection. Meniscus integrity and ligamentous stability are required, and any opposing chondral surface defects should be no greater than ICRS grade 2 [8]. Furthermore, osteotomies are often required to improve the success of the operation in patients with malalignment or patellofemoral defects [8, 58].

ACI has been investigated for use in the patient with early OA [59]. Minas *et al.* found that 92% of patients (mean age 38.3) had improvements in pain and function as long as 5 years after undergoing ACI for early OA defects of mean size 4.9 cm^2. Only 8% of patients went on to arthroplasty during the study period [59]. Niemeyer *et al.* performed a cohort study that compared ACI in patients younger than 40 to patients older than 40 and found that there were no differences in clinical results at 24 months postoperatively [60].

Advantages of ACI include the ability to produce durable hyaline-like cartilage in large (>2cm^2) defects. Disadvantages include the cost and complexity of two surgical procedures, the concern of de-differentiation of chondrocytes during expansion [61], and the risk of graft hypertrophy (which is highest with first-generation techniques). Additionally, first and second-generation techniques require an open arthrotomy, but this disadvantage is not associated with MACI.

STEM CELL THERAPY

Given that ACI requires two stages and that cultured chondrocytes de-differentiate, investigators have considered using mesenchymal stem cells (MSC) for cartilage regeneration [61, 62]. The first use of MSC in the treatment of a cartilage defect was in 1998 [63]. A recent review demonstrated that MSC use as part of a tissue-engineering strategy for the treatment of traumatic cartilage defects holds promise, but further investigation is required before protocols can be established [62]. Questions surrounding MSC source, and how best to culture and ultimately implant an MSC-seeded scaffold remain under investigation [62].

Likewise, stem cell therapy for the treatment of knee OA remains in the developmental stage. Like traumatic defects, OA defects may be amenable to treatment with an MSC-seeded scaffold, but this remains unknown [64]. An alternative strategy involves direct intra-articular injection of MSC. This technique has been reported by multiple authors with encouraging early results, but long-term, controlled studies are needed before conclusions can be made about its efficacy [65, 66].

A recent randomized controlled study investigated MSC as an adjunct to HTO and microfracture [67]. The group that received an MSC injection 3 weeks after surgery was found to have significantly better short-term functional scores and MRI findings than the group that received a hyaluronic acid injection 3 weeks postoperatively. Currently, it is difficult to know if injections alone are able to restore cartilage integrity for focal defects.

Proposed advantages of MSC therapy include negating the need for chondrocyte harvesting when used as part of a tissue engineering strategy, and its relative minimal invasiveness, when used as an intra-articular injection. The greatest disadvantage to MSC therapy at this time has to do with its experimental nature. Substantial further research is required before MSC therapy can be considered a viable treatment option in the management of knee OA.

AUTHORS' APPROACH

The authors' approach to early arthritic cartilage defects parallels the approach to other focal chondral defects (Fig. 1) [8]. Prerequisites to cartilage surgery include stability, proper alignment, and functional menisci. These factors may need to be addressed in conjunction with cartilage surgery. The following approach pertains to solitary full-thickness lesions with an intact peripheral rim that are isolated to one compartment. Cartilage loss involving all three compartments, unicompartmental disease with kissing lesions, or single lesions that lack an intact peripheral rim of normal cartilage may not be amenable to cartilage restoration surgery, and may be better treated with arthroplasty.

Patients with lower activity levels or factors that limit their ability to comply with postoperative rehabilitation protocols are less likely to be offered advanced cartilage repair techniques and are more likely to be treated with microfracture.

Small lesions ($<2cm^2$) are generally amenable to microfracture, provided that the depth of the lesion is less than 10 mm, and that there is no subchondral bone involvement. In small lesions that involve the subchondral bone, a single or double OATS plug is often recommended. If more than 2 OATS plugs are required to fill a defect (lesion usually >2cm2), the authors prefer using an osteochondral allograft.

In large lesions ($>2cm^2$), the authors are more likely to consider ACI/MACI or osteochondral allograft. ACI/MACI is the preferred technique for patellofemoral lesions, and it will typically be combined with an unloading tibial tubercle osteotomy if indicated. In patients with large defects of the femoral condyles with bone involvement, OCA is a viable option.

In smokers, the author has a direct discussion with the patient and advises him to quit smoking. A recent systematic review has shown poor outcomes after knee ligament and cartilage restorative procedures in smokers [68]. Even though all restorative procedures are affected negatively by smoking, the use of OCA in smokers is particularly cautioned against.

Rehabilitation is an integral component of cartilage surgery and is dictated in part by the location of the lesion. All lesions are treated with 6-8 hours of continuous passive motion per day, which has been shown to provide an optimal environment for cartilage repair [15]. Condylar lesions are protected by restricting weight-bearing, and patellofemoral lesions are protected by restricting knee flexion. In general, lesions are protected for approximately 6 weeks, but this may vary depending on the size of the defect relative to the size of the knee.

CASE STUDIES WITH ILLUSTRATIONS

Case 1:

A 51-year-old male had left knee pain for 5 years with no history of injury. He had previous hyaluronic acid injections without benefit. He enjoys hiking and would like to resume training for mountain climbing expedition. Examination of his left knee revealed no effusion, full range of motion, normal alignment, normal stability, and medial joint line tenderness. Plain films revealed minimal joint space narrowing (Fig. **2**). MRI revealed a small full-thickness cartilage defect with underlying bone edema (Fig. **3A,B**). Given ongoing symptoms and failure of conservative measures the patient was treated with an OATS procedure (Fig. **3C,D**).

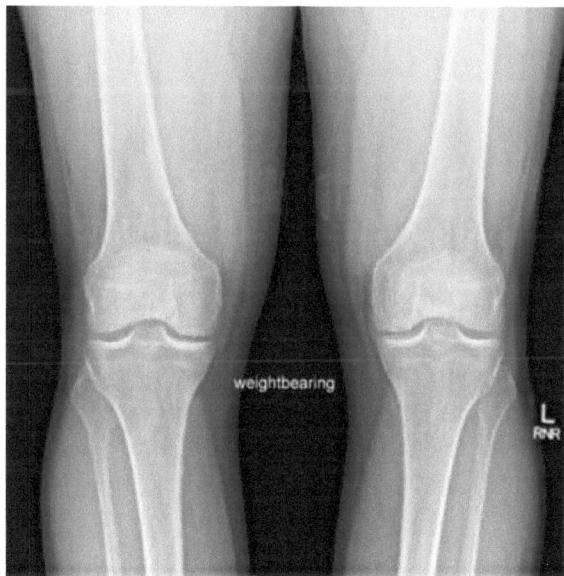

Fig. (2). Case 1: Radiograph of bilateral knees showing no significant joint space narrowing.

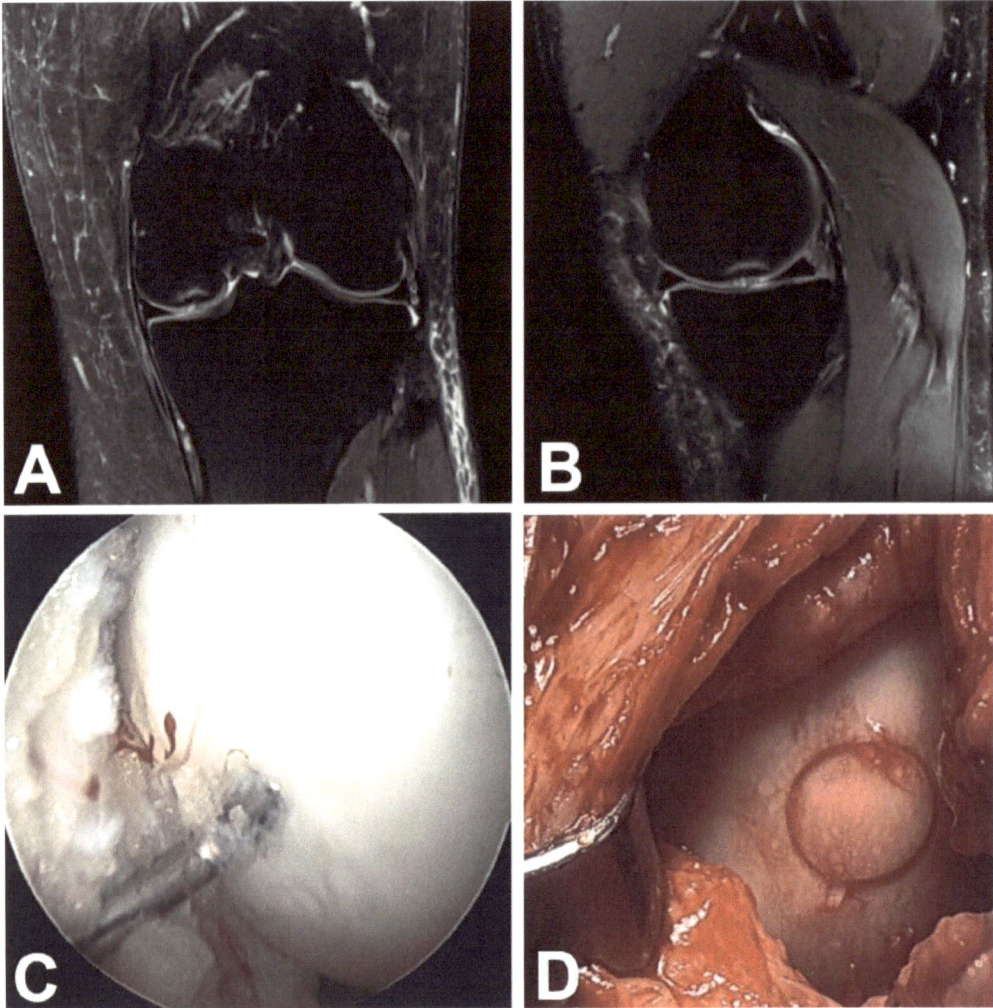

Fig. (3). Case 1: Coronal T2 MRI image (**A**) showing full thickness cartilage defect of medial femoral condyle. Sagittal T2 MRI image (**B**) showing cartilage defect of medial femoral condyle. Cartilage defect of medial femoral condyle (**C**) at time of arthroscopy. Cartilage defect of medial femoral condyle (**D**) after debridement.

Case 2:

A 53-year-old female nurse had chronic right knee pain, recurrent effusions and mechanical symptoms. She had previously undergone left TKR. On examination of her right knee, she was noted to have a small effusion, full range of motion, normal alignment, normal stability and tenderness of the lateral joint line. Plain films were unremarkable (Fig. **4A**). MRI revealed a medium sized full-thickness cartilage defect of the lateral femoral condyle (Fig. **4B,C**). The isolated defect of the lateral femoral condyle was measured to be 2.2 cm x 1.2 cm. Given ongoing symptoms and failure of conservative measures, as well as a BMI >30, the patient was treated with microfracture (Fig. **4D-F**).

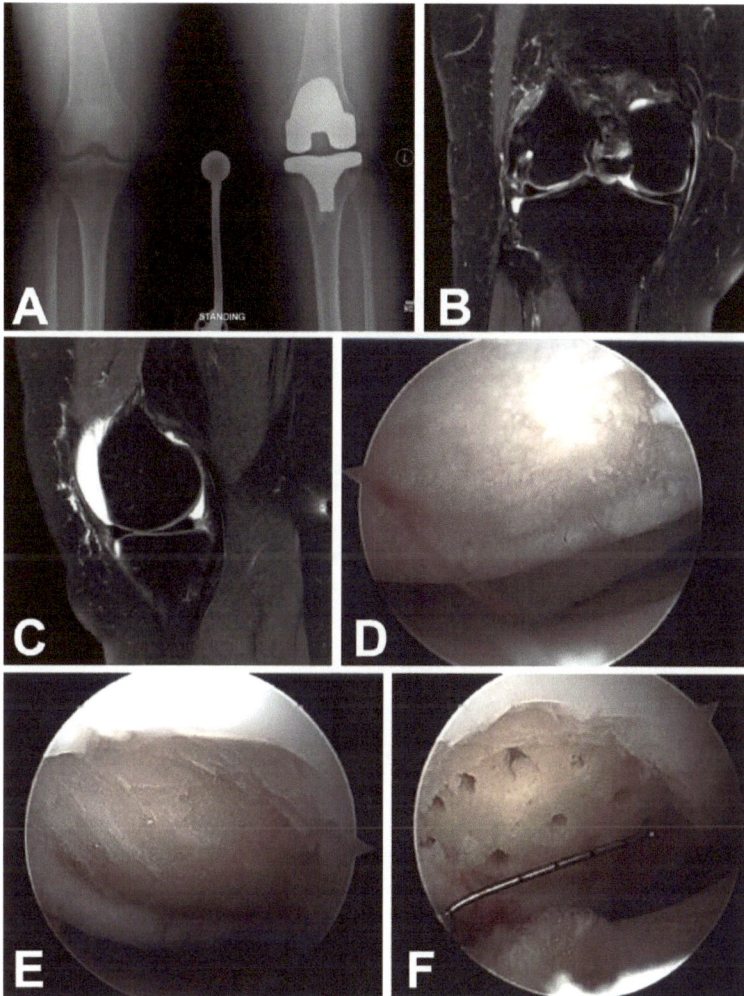

Fig. (4). Case 2: Radiograph (**A**) of bilateral knees showing no significant joint space narrowing. Coronal T2 MRI image (**B**) showing full thickness cartilage defect of lateral femoral condyle. Sagittal T2 MRI image (**C**) showing cartilage defect of lateral femoral condyle. Cartilage defect (**D**) of lateral femoral condyle at time of arthroscopy. Cartilage defect (**E**) of lateral femoral condyle after debridement. Cartilage defect (**F**) of lateral femoral condyle after microfracture.

CONCLUSION

Cartilage surgery is a treatment option in a subset of early OA patients. Decisions regarding which technique to employ should be made on a case-by-case basis. Both patient and lesion-specific factors must be considered before offering surgery of this type. Patients must be educated about expectations and motivated to participate in post-operative rehabilitation before any cartilage surgery. Having an understanding of available cartilage surgeries will assist clinicians as they counsel patients with early knee OA.

CONFLICT OF INTEREST

The authors confirm that the author have no conflict of interest to declare for this publication.

ACKNOWLEDGEMENTS

Declared none.

REFERENCES

[1]   Buckwalter JA, Mankin HJ. Articular cartilage: tissue design and chondrocyte-matrix interactions. Instr Course Lect 1998; 47: 477-86.
        [PMID: 9571449]

[2]   Buckwalter JA, Mankin HJ. Articular cartilage. 2. Degeneration and osteoarthrosis, repair, regeneration, and transplantation. J Bone Joint Surg Am 1997; 79A(4): 612-32.

[3]   Lawrence RC, Felson DT, Helmick CG, *et al.* Estimates of the prevalence of arthritis and other rheumatic conditions in the United States. Part II. Arthritis Rheum 2008; 58(1): 26-35.
        [http://dx.doi.org/10.1002/art.23176] [PMID: 18163497]

[4]   Felson DT. Clinical practice. Osteoarthritis of the knee. N Engl J Med 2006; 354(8): 841-8.
        [http://dx.doi.org/10.1056/NEJMcp051726] [PMID: 16495396]

[5]   Messner K, Maletius W. The long-term prognosis for severe damage to weight-bearing cartilage in the knee: a 14-year clinical and radiographic follow-up in 28 young athletes. Acta Orthop Scand 1996; 67(2): 165-8.
        [http://dx.doi.org/10.3109/17453679608994664] [PMID: 8623573]

[6]   Widuchowski W, Widuchowski J, Trzaska T. Articular cartilage defects: study of 25,124 knee arthroscopies. Knee 2007; 14(3): 177-82.
        [http://dx.doi.org/10.1016/j.knee.2007.02.001] [PMID: 17428666]

[7]   Bijlsma JW, Berenbaum F, Lafeber FP. Osteoarthritis: an update with relevance for clinical practice. Lancet 2011; 377(9783): 2115-26.

[http://dx.doi.org/10.1016/S0140-6736(11)60243-2] [PMID: 21684382]

[8]   Cole BJ, Pascual-Garrido C, Grumet RC. Surgical management of articular cartilage defects in the knee. J Bone Joint Surg Am 2009; 91(7): 1778-90.
        [PMID: 19571102]

[9]   Farr J, Cole B, Dhawan A, Kercher J, Sherman S. Clinical cartilage restoration: evolution and overview. Clin Orthop Relat Res 2011; 469(10): 2696-705.
        [http://dx.doi.org/10.1007/s11999-010-1764-z] [PMID: 21240578]

[10]   Alford JW, Cole BJ. Cartilage restoration, part 1: basic science, historical perspective, patient evaluation, and treatment options. Am J Sports Med 2005; 33(2): 295-306.
        [http://dx.doi.org/10.1177/0363546504273510] [PMID: 15701618]

[11]   Alford JW, Cole BJ. Cartilage restoration, part 2: techniques, outcomes, and future directions. Am J Sports Med 2005; 33(3): 443-60.
        [http://dx.doi.org/10.1177/0363546505274578] [PMID: 15716263]

[12]   Behery O, Siston RA, Harris JD, Flanigan DC. Treatment of cartilage defects of the knee: expanding on the existing algorithm. Clin J Sport Med 2014; 24(1): 21-30.
        [http://dx.doi.org/10.1097/JSM.0000000000000004] [PMID: 24157464]

[13]   Gudas R, Gudaite A, Pocius A, *et al.* Ten-year follow-up of a prospective, randomized clinical study of mosaic osteochondral autologous transplantation *versus* microfracture for the treatment of osteochondral defects in the knee joint of athletes. Am J Sports Med 2012; 40(11): 2499-508.
        [http://dx.doi.org/10.1177/0363546512458763] [PMID: 23024150]

[14]   Knutsen G, Drogset JO, Engebretsen L, *et al.* A randomized trial comparing autologous chondrocyte implantation with microfracture. Findings at five years. J Bone Joint Surg Am 2007; 89(10): 2105-12.
        [http://dx.doi.org/10.2106/JBJS.G.00003] [PMID: 17908884]

[15]   Steadman JR, Rodkey WG, Briggs KK. Microfracture chondroplasty: Indications, techniques, and outcomes. Sports Med Arthrosc Rev 2003; 11(4): 236-44.
        [http://dx.doi.org/10.1097/00132585-200311040-00004]

[16]   Steadman JR, Rodkey WG, Singleton SB, Briggs KK. Microfracture technique for full-thickness chondral defects: Technique and clinical results. Oper Tech Orthop 1997; 7(4): 300-4.
        [http://dx.doi.org/10.1016/S1048-6666(97)80033-X]

[17]   Buckwalter JA, Lohmander S. Operative treatment of osteoarthrosis. Current practice and future development. J Bone Joint Surg Am 1994; 76(9): 1405-18.
        [PMID: 8077274]

[18]   Honig K, Vidal A, McCarty E. Microfracture. Tech Knee Surg 2009; 8(1): 7-13.
        [http://dx.doi.org/10.1097/BTK.0b013e31819b2f2d]

[19]   Chen H, Sun J, Hoemann CD, *et al.* Drilling and microfracture lead to different bone structure and necrosis during bone-marrow stimulation for cartilage repair. J Orthop Res 2009; 27(11): 1432-8.
        [http://dx.doi.org/10.1002/jor.20905] [PMID: 19402150]

[20]   Goyal D, Goyal A, Keyhani S, Lee EH, Hui JH. Evidence-based status of second- and third-generation autologous chondrocyte implantation over first generation: a systematic review of level I and II studies. Arthroscopy 2013; 29(11): 1872-8.

[http://dx.doi.org/10.1016/j.arthro.2013.07.271] [PMID: 24075851]

[21]   Mithoefer K, McAdams T, Williams RJ, Kreuz PC, Mandelbaum BR. Clinical efficacy of the microfracture technique for articular cartilage repair in the knee: an evidence-based systematic analysis. Am J Sports Med 2009; 37(10): 2053-63.
[http://dx.doi.org/10.1177/0363546508328414] [PMID: 19251676]

[22]   Steadman JR, Briggs KK, Rodrigo JJ, Kocher MS, Gill TJ, Rodkey WG. Outcomes of microfracture for traumatic chondral defects of the knee: average 11-year follow-up. Arthroscopy 2003; 19(5): 477-84.
[http://dx.doi.org/10.1053/jars.2003.50112] [PMID: 12724676]

[23]   Miller BS, Steadman JR, Briggs KK, Rodrigo JJ, Rodkey WG. Patient satisfaction and outcome after microfracture of the degenerative knee. J Knee Surg 2004; 17(1): 13-7.
[PMID: 14971668]

[24]   Bae DK, Yoon KH, Song SJ. Cartilage healing after microfracture in osteoarthritic knees. Arthroscopy 2006; 22(4): 367-74.
[http://dx.doi.org/10.1016/j.arthro.2006.01.015] [PMID: 16581448]

[25]   Steadman JR, Ramappa AJ, Maxwell RB, Briggs KK. An arthroscopic treatment regimen for osteoarthritis of the knee. Arthroscopy 2007; 23(9): 948-55.
[http://dx.doi.org/10.1016/j.arthro.2007.03.097] [PMID: 17868833]

[26]   Bae DK, Song SJ, Yoon KH, Heo DB, Kim TJ. Survival analysis of microfracture in the osteoarthritic knee-minimum 10-year follow-up. Arthroscopy 2013; 29(2): 244-50.
[http://dx.doi.org/10.1016/j.arthro.2012.09.006] [PMID: 23369477]

[27]   Sakata K, Furumatsu T, Abe N, Miyazawa S, Sakoma Y, Ozaki T. Histological analysis of failed cartilage repair after marrow stimulation for the treatment of large cartilage defect in medial compartmental osteoarthritis of the knee. Acta Med Okayama 2013; 67(1): 65-74.
[PMID: 23439511]

[28]   Kaul G, Cucchiarini M, Remberger K, Kohn D, Madry H. Failed cartilage repair for early osteoarthritis defects: a biochemical, histological and immunohistochemical analysis of the repair tissue after treatment with marrow-stimulation techniques. Knee Surg Sports Traumatol Arthrosc 2012; 20(11): 2315-24.
[http://dx.doi.org/10.1007/s00167-011-1853-x] [PMID: 22222614]

[29]   Sterett WI, Steadman JR, Huang MJ, Matheny LM, Briggs KK. Chondral resurfacing and high tibial osteotomy in the varus knee: survivorship analysis. Am J Sports Med 2010; 38(7): 1420-4.
[http://dx.doi.org/10.1177/0363546509360403] [PMID: 20375366]

[30]   Miller BS, Joseph TA, Barry EM, Rich VJ, Sterett WI. Patient satisfaction after medial opening high tibial osteotomy and microfracture. J Knee Surg 2007; 20(2): 129-33.
[PMID: 17486904]

[31]   Matsunaga D, Akizuki S, Takizawa T, Yamazaki I, Kuraishi J. Repair of articular cartilage and clinical outcome after osteotomy with microfracture or abrasion arthroplasty for medial gonarthrosis. Knee 2007; 14(6): 465-71.
[http://dx.doi.org/10.1016/j.knee.2007.06.008] [PMID: 17822904]

[32] Lee GW, Son JH, Kim JD, Jung GH. Is platelet-rich plasma able to enhance the results of arthroscopic microfracture in early osteoarthritis and cartilage lesion over 40 years of age? Eur J Orthop Surg Traumatol 2013; 23(5): 581-7.
[http://dx.doi.org/10.1007/s00590-012-1038-4] [PMID: 23412171]

[33] Gille J, Behrens P, Volpi P, *et al.* Outcome of Autologous Matrix Induced Chondrogenesis (AMIC) in cartilage knee surgery: data of the AMIC Registry. Arch Orthop Trauma Surg 2013; 133(1): 87-93.
[http://dx.doi.org/10.1007/s00402-012-1621-5] [PMID: 23070222]

[34] Gille J, Schuseil E, Wimmer J, Gellissen J, Schulz AP, Behrens P. Mid-term results of Autologous Matrix-Induced Chondrogenesis for treatment of focal cartilage defects in the knee. Knee Surg Sports Traumatol Arthrosc 2010; 18(11): 1456-64.
[http://dx.doi.org/10.1007/s00167-010-1042-3] [PMID: 20127072]

[35] Schiavone Panni A, Cerciello S, Vasso M. The management of knee cartilage defects with modified amic technique: preliminary results. Int J Immunopathol Pharmacol 2011; 24(1) (Suppl. 2): 149-52.
[PMID: 21669155]

[36] Benthien JP, Behrens P. The treatment of chondral and osteochondral defects of the knee with autologous matrix-induced chondrogenesis (AMIC): method description and recent developments. Knee Surg Sports Traumatol Arthrosc 2011; 19(8): 1316-9.
[http://dx.doi.org/10.1007/s00167-010-1356-1] [PMID: 21234543]

[37] Steinwachs MR, Guggi T, Kreuz PC. Marrow stimulation techniques. Injury 2008; 39 (Suppl. 1): S26-31.
[http://dx.doi.org/10.1016/j.injury.2008.01.042] [PMID: 18313469]

[38] Anders S, Volz M, Frick H, Gellissen J. A randomized, controlled trial comparing autologous matrix-induced chondrogenesis (AMIC®) to microfracture: Analysis of 1- and 2-year follow-up data of 2 centers. Open Orthop J 2013; 7: 133-43.
[http://dx.doi.org/10.2174/1874325001307010133] [PMID: 23730377]

[39] Hangody L, Kish G, Kárpáti Z, Udvarhelyi I, Szigeti I, Bély M. Mosaicplasty for the treatment of articular cartilage defects: application in clinical practice. Orthopedics 1998; 21(7): 751-6.
[PMID: 9672912]

[40] Bobic V, Morgan CD, Carter T. Osteochondral autologous graft transfer. Oper Tech Sports Med 2000; 8(2): 168-78.
[http://dx.doi.org/10.1053/otsm.2000.7506]

[41] Hangody L, Füles P. Autologous osteochondral mosaicplasty for the treatment of full-thickness defects of weight-bearing joints: ten years of experimental and clinical experience. J Bone Joint Surg Am 2003; 85-A (Suppl. 2): 25-32.
[PMID: 12721342]

[42] Gudas R, Kalesinskas RJ, Kimtys V, *et al.* A prospective randomized clinical study of mosaic osteochondral autologous transplantation *versus* microfracture for the treatment of osteochondral defects in the knee joint in young athletes. Arthroscopy 2005; 21(9): 1066-75.
[http://dx.doi.org/10.1016/j.arthro.2005.06.018] [PMID: 16171631]

[43] Bentley G, Biant LC, Carrington RW, *et al.* A prospective, randomised comparison of autologous

chondrocyte implantation *versus* mosaicplasty for osteochondral defects in the knee. J Bone Joint Surg Br 2003; 85(2): 223-30.
[http://dx.doi.org/10.1302/0301-620X.85B2.13543] [PMID: 12678357]

[44]   Dozin B, Malpeli M, Cancedda R, *et al.* Comparative evaluation of autologous chondrocyte implantation and mosaicplasty: a multicentered randomized clinical trial. Clin J Sport Med 2005; 15(4): 220-6.
[http://dx.doi.org/10.1097/01.jsm.0000171882.66432.80] [PMID: 16003035]

[45]   Horas U, Pelinkovic D, Herr G, Aigner T, Schnettler R. Autologous chondrocyte implantation and osteochondral cylinder transplantation in cartilage repair of the knee joint. A prospective, comparative trial. J Bone Joint Surg Am 2003; 85-A(2): 185-92.
[PMID: 12571292]

[46]   Andres BM, Mears SC, Somel DS, Klug R, Wenz JF. Treatment of osteoarthritic cartilage lesions with osteochondral autograft transplantation. Orthopedics 2003; 26(11): 1121-6.
[PMID: 14627109]

[47]   Garrett JC. Treatment of osteochondral defects of the distal femur with fresh osteochondral allografts: a preliminary report. Arthroscopy 1986; 2(4): 222-6.
[http://dx.doi.org/10.1016/S0749-8063(86)80076-7] [PMID: 3801101]

[48]   Gross AE, Silverstein EA, Falk J, Falk R, Langer F. The allotransplantation of partial joints in the treatment of osteoarthritis of the knee. Clin Orthop Relat Res 1975; (108): 7-14.
[http://dx.doi.org/10.1097/00003086-197505000-00003] [PMID: 1139838]

[49]   Bugbee W, Cavallo M, Giannini S. Osteochondral allograft transplantation in the knee. J Knee Surg 2012; 25(2): 109-16.
[http://dx.doi.org/10.1055/s-0032-1313743] [PMID: 22928428]

[50]   Gross AE, Kim W, Las Heras F, Backstein D, Safir O, Pritzker KP. Fresh osteochondral allografts for posttraumatic knee defects: long-term followup. Clin Orthop Relat Res 2008; 466(8): 1863-70.
[http://dx.doi.org/10.1007/s11999-008-0282-8] [PMID: 18465182]

[51]   Meyers MH, Akeson W, Convery FR. Resurfacing of the knee with fresh osteochondral allograft. J Bone Joint Surg Am 1989; 71(5): 704-13.
[PMID: 2659599]

[52]   McDermott AG, Langer F, Pritzker KP, Gross AE. Fresh small-fragment osteochondral allografts. Long-term follow-up study on first 100 cases. Clin Orthop Relat Res 1985; (197): 96-102.
[PMID: 3893835]

[53]   Brittberg M, Lindahl A, Nilsson A, Ohlsson C, Isaksson O, Peterson L. Treatment of deep cartilage defects in the knee with autologous chondrocyte transplantation. N Engl J Med 1994; 331(14): 889-95.
[http://dx.doi.org/10.1056/NEJM199410063311401] [PMID: 8078550]

[54]   Peterson L, Minas T, Brittberg M, Nilsson A, Sjögren-Jansson E, Lindahl A. Two- to 9-year outcome after autologous chondrocyte transplantation of the knee. Clin Orthop Relat Res 2000; (374): 212-34.
[http://dx.doi.org/10.1097/00003086-200005000-00020] [PMID: 10818982]

[55]   Gomoll AH, Probst C, Farr J, Cole BJ, Minas T. Use of a type I/III bilayer collagen membrane decreases reoperation rates for symptomatic hypertrophy after autologous chondrocyte implantation.

Am J Sports Med 2009; 37 (Suppl. 1): 20S-3S.
[http://dx.doi.org/10.1177/0363546509348477] [PMID: 19841142]

[56] Steinwachs M. New technique for cell-seeded collagen-matrix-supported autologous chondrocyte transplantation. Arthroscopy 2009; 25(2): 208-11.
[http://dx.doi.org/10.1016/j.arthro.2008.10.009] [PMID: 19171282]

[57] Peterson L, Vasiliadis HS, Brittberg M, Lindahl A. Autologous chondrocyte implantation: a long-term follow-up. Am J Sports Med 2010; 38(6): 1117-24.
[http://dx.doi.org/10.1177/0363546509357915] [PMID: 20181804]

[58] Trinh TQ, Harris JD, Siston RA, Flanigan DC. Improved outcomes with combined autologous chondrocyte implantation and patellofemoral osteotomy *versus* isolated autologous chondrocyte implantation. Arthroscopy 2013; 29(3): 566-74.
[http://dx.doi.org/10.1016/j.arthro.2012.10.008] [PMID: 23312875]

[59] Minas T, Gomoll AH, Solhpour S, Rosenberger R, Probst C, Bryant T. Autologous chondrocyte implantation for joint preservation in patients with early osteoarthritis. Clin Orthop Relat Res 2010; 468(1): 147-57.
[http://dx.doi.org/10.1007/s11999-009-0998-0] [PMID: 19653049]

[60] Niemeyer P, Köstler W, Salzmann GM, Lenz P, Kreuz PC, Südkamp NP. Autologous chondrocyte implantation for treatment of focal cartilage defects in patients age 40 years and older: A matched-pair analysis with 2-year follow-up. Am J Sports Med 2010; 38(12): 2410-6.
[http://dx.doi.org/10.1177/0363546510376742] [PMID: 20829417]

[61] von der Mark K, Gauss V, von der Mark H, Müller P. Relationship between cell shape and type of collagen synthesised as chondrocytes lose their cartilage phenotype in culture. Nature 1977; 267(5611): 531-2.
[http://dx.doi.org/10.1038/267531a0] [PMID: 559947]

[62] Bornes TD, Adesida AB, Jomha NM. Mesenchymal stem cells in the treatment of traumatic articular cartilage defects: a comprehensive review. Arthritis Res Ther 2014; 16(5): 432.
[http://dx.doi.org/10.1186/s13075-014-0432-1] [PMID: 25606595]

[63] Wakitani S, Mitsuoka T, Nakamura N, Toritsuka Y, Nakamura Y, Horibe S. Autologous bone marrow stromal cell transplantation for repair of full-thickness articular cartilage defects in human patellae: two case reports. Cell Transplant 2004; 13(5): 595-600.
[http://dx.doi.org/10.3727/000000004783983747] [PMID: 15565871]

[64] Diekman BO, Guilak F. Stem cell-based therapies for osteoarthritis: challenges and opportunities. Curr Opin Rheumatol 2013; 25(1): 119-26.
[http://dx.doi.org/10.1097/BOR.0b013e32835aa28d] [PMID: 23190869]

[65] Orozco L, Munar A, Soler R, *et al.* Treatment of knee osteoarthritis with autologous mesenchymal stem cells: a pilot study. Transplantation 2013; 95(12): 1535-41.
[http://dx.doi.org/10.1097/TP.0b013e318291a2da] [PMID: 23680930]

[66] Jo CH, Lee YG, Shin WH, *et al.* Intra-articular injection of mesenchymal stem cells for the treatment of osteoarthritis of the knee: a proof-of-concept clinical trial. Stem Cells 2014; 32(5): 1254-66.
[http://dx.doi.org/10.1002/stem.1634] [PMID: 24449146]

[67]   Wong KL, Lee KB, Tai BC, Law P, Lee EH, Hui JH. Injectable cultured bone marrow-derived mesenchymal stem cells in varus knees with cartilage defects undergoing high tibial osteotomy: a prospective, randomized controlled clinical trial with 2 years follow-up. Arthroscopy 2013; 29(12): 2020-8.
        [http://dx.doi.org/10.1016/j.arthro.2013.09.074] [PMID: 24286801]

[68]   Kanneganti P, Harris JD, Brophy RH, Carey JL, Lattermann C, Flanigan DC. The effect of smoking on ligament and cartilage surgery in the knee: a systematic review. Am J Sports Med 2012; 40(12): 2872-8.
        [http://dx.doi.org/10.1177/0363546512458223] [PMID: 22972849]

CHAPTER 7

Opening Wedge Osteotomies of the Proximal Tibia and Distal Femur

Maurizio Montalti[1,2] and **Saverio Affatato**[2,*]

[1] *Orthopaedic-Traumatology and Prosthetic surgery and revisions of hip and knee implants, Rizzoli Orthopaedic Institute, Bologna-Italy*

[2] *Medical Technology Laboratory, Rizzoli Orthopaedic Institute, Bologna-Italy*

Abstract: The use of osteotomy is a method to restore knee alignment and is based on the transfer of weight-bearing forces from the area affected by arthrosis to a healthy region of the knee. This force redistribution is the distinctive aspect of osteotomy when compared to other treatment methods. In the last decades, since the introduction and success of knee arthroplasty, the predominance of osteotomy has gradually declined. Nowadays, the actual necessity of osteotomy, beside as a prophylactic operation, is still debated. However, osteotomy remains a valuable technique, in agreement with precise patient indications.

Keywords: Biomechanics, Lateral opening wedge, Medial opening wedge, Osteotomy, Osteotomy contraindications, Patient selection, Postoperative axis, Postoperative rehabilitation, Preoperative axis, Radiographic evaluation, Surgical procedure.

INTRODUCTION

Knee osteotomy is a surgical procedure that may be recommended when arthritis damage is observed in confined to one area of the knee joint. The procedure consists of removing or adding a wedge of bone to the proximal tibia or lower femur to help shift your body weight off the damaged portion of your knee joint

* **Corresponding author Saverio Affatato:** Medical Technology Laboratory, Rizzoli Orthopaedic Institute, Bologna-Italy; Tel: +39-51-6366865; Fax: +39-51-6366863; E-mail: affatato@tecno.ior.it

(Fig. **1**). Knee osteotomy is performed on people who may be considered too young for a total knee replacement.

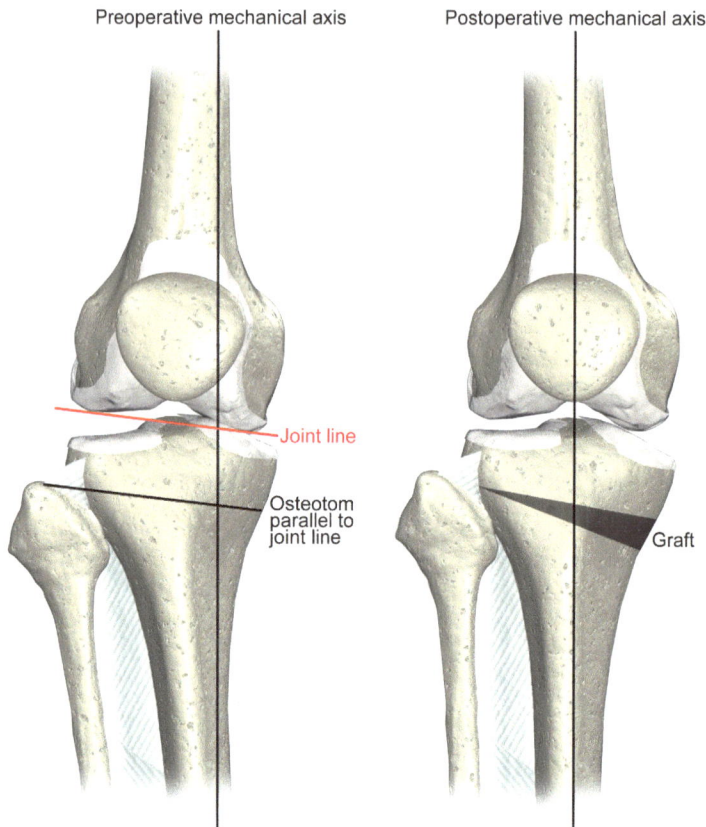

Fig. (1). Preoperative mechanical axis and postoperative mechanical axis (Medial opening wedge proximal tibial osteotomy).

Because prosthetic knees may wear out over time, an osteotomy procedure can enable younger, active osteoarthritis patients to continue using the healthy portion of their knee. The procedure can delay the need for a total knee replacement for up to ten years. In the last decades, since the introduction and success of knee arthroplasty, the predominance of osteotomy has gradually declined. Nowadays, the actual necessity of osteotomy, beside as a prophylactic operation, is still debated. Osteotomy is an efficient surgical technique if used with precise patient indications. Osteotomy can present many complications and adequate patient selection is mandatory to minimize major complications.

BIOMECHANICAL CONSIDERATION

During normal walking, a TKR is subjected to different joint loading conditions due to a number of highly demanding activities. *Load stress concentration, due to load transmission between the tibial and the femoral components, may have critical effects during daily living of the knee.* A simplification of these waveforms, derived from fluoroscopic analyses is showed in Fig. (**2**).

Axial load under HDDA

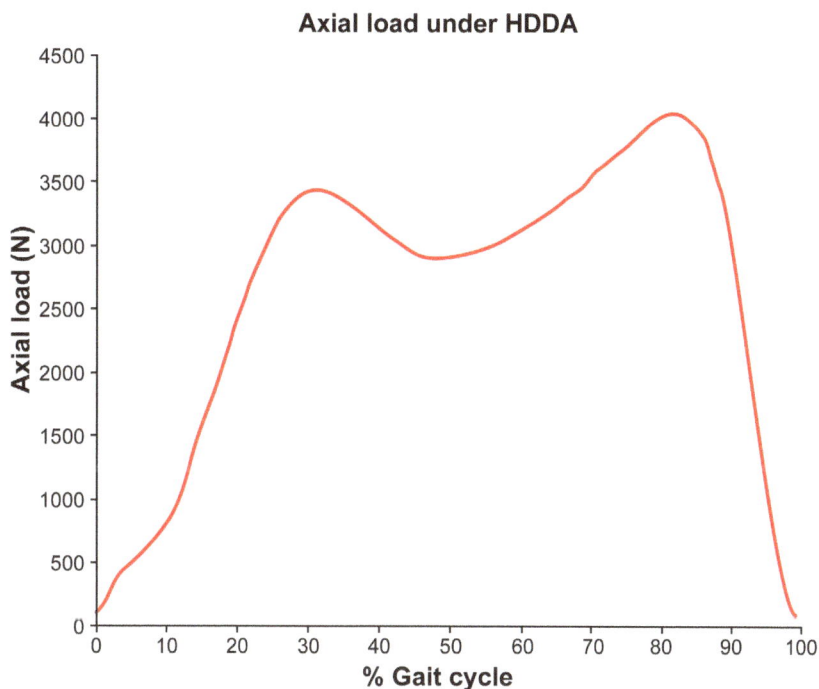

Fig. (2). A simplification of the axial load derived from fluoroscopic analyses.

The first peak is caused by the large quadriceps tension that is necessary to arrest the descent of the body mass, when the weight transfers from the leg that is pushing off from the ground, to the leg that is accepting the load shortly after the heel strikes the ground. This force curve includes a second peak, when the knee and hip are extended, the heel is raised from the floor and the forefoot is pushing off, propelling the body forwards [1]. Osteoarthrosis commonly arises when biological resistance is not able to bear mechanical stressing and excessive pressure on articular surface [2]. This loss of force balance causes, as a start, a surface deformity, followed by the development of osteoarthrosis. Joint stability is a result of the equilibrium between two forces; active muscular forces and passive ligamentous forces have to balance the force eccentrically exerted by the part of the body supported by the knee.

The tibio-femoral articular geometry is adapted to the gait-loading pattern. When each of the medial and lateral compartments is sectioned in the sagittal plane, the medial is seen to be more congruent: the femoral condyle rests in a shallow concavity in the tibial plateau [1]. Conversely, the lateral femoral condyle bears onto a flat or even convex contour, which implies a much smaller articular contact area and, hence, higher contact stresses if the forces are similar to those in the medial compartment. A corollary of this morphology is that a lateral meniscectomy has a larger effect on the contact stresses than does a medial one [3]. The consequence of the peak joint force falling on the medial compartment is that, despite the morphological adaptation, it is the most common site of degenerative changes.

Studies have demonstrated that during the gait cycle, people with knee osteoarthritis and varus alignment walk with specific knee biomechanics and muscular function [4, 5]. In particular, an increased knee adduction moment is typically observed in patients with medial knee osteoarthritis and has also been associated with accelerated disease progression [6].

The principal advantages of opening wedge high tibial osteotomy include maintenance of the bone stock, correction of the deformity close to its origin, and no requirement for a fibular osteotomy [7, 8]. The biomechanical principle of high tibial osteotomy in medial compartment OA is to redistribute the weight bearing forces from the worn medial compartment towards the lateral compartment to relieve pain and to slow disease progression [9, 10]. This can be accompanied by pain relief and improvements in gait and function.

The structure and mechanical properties of a particular bone, also reflected by its bone mineral density, correspond to the stresses it must bear. In pathological condition of osteoarthritis, there is an increase of the ratio between medial condyle and lateral condyle mineral densities [2].

Indications and Patients Selection

The patient selection is crucial in achieving a successful surgical procedure. In the last years total knee arthroplasty represents a viable alternative of the osteotomy and therefore selection criteria have became more restrictive.

Some conditions predispose to poor outcomes of the osteotomy and these include: advanced age (patients over the age of 60) [11, 12], severe arthritic changes [13], patella-femoral arthrosis, limited articular range of motion, angular knee deformities (Varus knee > 10° and valgus knee > 15°) ([14], lateral tibial subluxation more than 1 cm, knee flexion contracture > 15°, inflammatory arthritis and chondrocalcinosis. Angular deformities that exceed previous values are often associated with significant ligamentous laxity that represents a contraindication for osteotomy. Relative contraindications are: body weight > 90 Kg and patients presenting with patella Baja or Alta [15].

Osteotomy may be still *appropriate* for younger patient with unicompartimental arthritis. There is no general consensus about the meaning of the word "young"; Insall *et al.* [2] suggested performing osteotomy in patients younger than 55 to 60 years old. Moreover osteotomy is more suitable for patients with higher levels of activities that involve heavy works or high-demand sports; in these patients there is a potential risk of increased wear and premature failure of knee arthroplasty. There are many studies in the literature that compare UKA (unicompartmental knee arthroplasty) with high tibial osteotomy for the treatment of medial compartment knee osteoarthritis [16, 17]. Dettoni and coworkers [18] reported the clinical and radiological midterm results of 56 consecutive UKA and 54 Opening wedge HTO (high tibial osteotomy). They stated that the outcomes were comparable in the two groups. Patient with > 30% ideal body weight had a significantly greater risk for failure (recurrent pain and loss of correction). Inflammatory pathology, as rheumatoid arthritis, produces poor clinical results in high tibial osteotomy [19]. Also chondrocalcinosis significantly affects the long-term success of the surgical procedure [20].

Examination of the Patient and Radiographic Evaluation

Physical examination of the knee joint and lower limbs is basic in the selection of the appropriate patient. Insall *et al.* [2] stated that some aspects should be carefully examined: angular deformity, torsional pattern of the limb, position of the foot, presence of limp, flexion deformity and presence of varus thrust. Knee examination should include gait abnormalities during walking, range of motion, patella-femoral evaluation, presence or absence of subluxation of the femoral tibial articulation and varus-valgus instability. Knee instability should be checked to avoid under correction during the surgical procedure but moderate medial laxity does not contraindicate osteotomy and evidences of osteoarthritis and arterial insufficiency should be tested during the physical examination [2].

Radiographic evaluation helps the surgeon to plan the surgical procedure. The correct assessment of lower limb alignment is obtained by full standing radiographs. The knee might be flexed to approximately 5° to avoid the abnormal varus *recurvatum* position. Hip-knee-ankle angle radiographs allow us to determine if signs of overload are present and to confirm the indication of osteotomy. If the X-ray showed signs of wear or disease of the contralateral compartment, an inflammatory or a metabolic disease can be supposed and the indication of performing osteotomy may be questioned [2]. Furthermore radiographs focus the site of the osteotomy. The radiographic exam should include: antero-posterior and lateral radiographs with the patient in supine position and knee 5° flexed, hip-knee-ankle angle radiographs (alignment assessment) with the patient in bipodal standing.

The angle formed by the axes of the anatomical femur and tibia is the easiest method to measure the alignment of the limb. Usually this angle measures between 5 and 8° of valgus on a radiogram performed under load of the lower limb. The mechanical axis of the lower limb can be used to determine the size of the wedge. It is estimated that more or less every degree of the angle corresponds to 1 mm thickness of the bone wedge. Coventry *et al.* [19] described a valid method to plan a high tibial osteotomy. To stabilize the corrective wedge on preoperative radiographs we localize the centre of the femoral head and tibio-talar joint on the full standing radiographs. Then we identify and mark the selected weight-bearing-line on the tibial plateau that usually passes through the lateral tibio-femoral compartment (*about 60% of the width of the tibia*). The first line is drawn from the centre of the femoral head to the tibial plateau coordinate and a second line is drawn from the centre of the ankle joint to the tibial plateau coordinate. The angular correction required to realign the weight-bearing-line as desired is represented by the angle resulting from the two intersecting lines.

In our opinion the osteotomy should be tibial in varus knee and femoral in valgus knee even if some authors [19, 21] reported good results of tibial osteotomy performed on a moderate valgus knee (obliquity of the joint line not greater than 10°).

Surgical Technique for Medial Opening Wedge Proximal Tibial Osteotomy

The patient is placed supine with the tourniquet at the root of the lower limb. Preoperative antibiotics are administered. The incision is antero-medial between the tibial tubercle and the posteromedial border of the tibia. In the future the incision may be used through medial para-patellar approach if a total knee replacement will be necessary. A dissection of hamstring tendons and an exposition and separation from the bone (at the level of the osteotomy) of medial collateral ligament is performed. A periosteal elevator is used in order to retract the medial collateral ligament medially while the patellar tendon is retracted laterally. A guide pin is positioned starting at least 3, 5 cm distal to the medial tibial plateau and continuing laterally and proximally toward the tip of the fibula. The procedure is realized under fluoroscopic guidance and the orientation of the pin determines the angle of the osteotomy. After the fluoroscopic control of the position of the guide wire osteotomy is carried out opening the medial side, and keeping the lateral cortex intact. The osteotomy is started with oscillating saw (placed parallel to the guide pin) and is completed with thin osteotomy to increase accuracy and to avoid breakage of the lateral cortex. The cut ends approximately 1 cm before the lateral tibial cortex (Fig. **3**).

A valgus stress together with the use of larger osteotomies allows opening the osteotomy to the desired correction. A two-holed osteotomy plate (Puddu plate) is positioned into the osteotomy site and 4.5-cortical screws are placed through the holes. To fill the osseous gap a wedge shaped bone graft (allograft) is used. Bone graft is the best bone filling material because of its osteoconductive, osteoinductive and osteogenic properties [22].

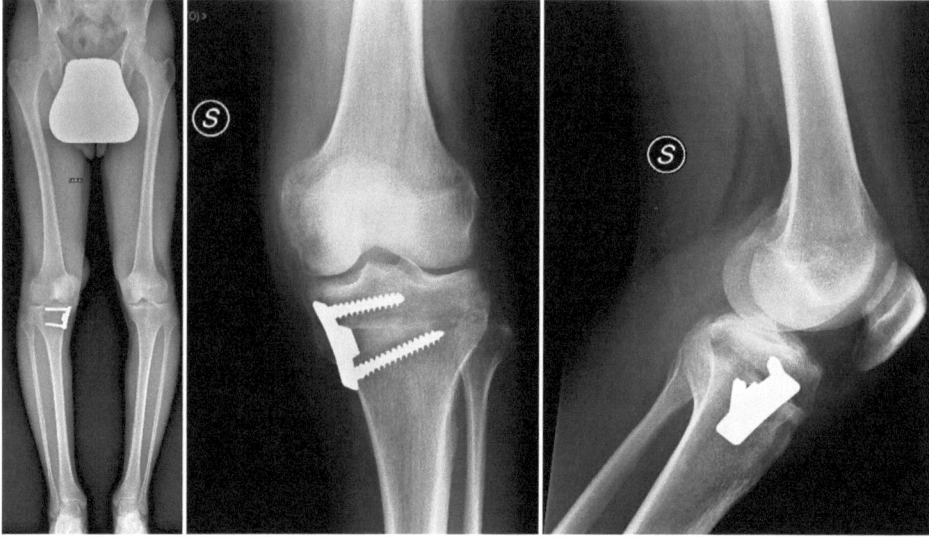

Fig. (3). Preoperative X-rays and postoperative X-rays (A-P view and L-L view) after medial opening wedge proximal tibial osteotomy.

The disadvantage of this technique are represented by the longer uniting time and by the need of varying amounts of bone grafts on the basis of the degree of correction to obtain.

Currently locking compression plates designed for stable fixation of the osteotomies are available on the market (Tomofix, Depuy-Synthes). The characteristics of these plates are the possibility to achieve dynamic compression and the improvement of screws retention in plate and in cortical bone due to the presence of multiple fixed-angles locking holes in the plate.

Medial opening wedge osteotomy has several advantages over a lateral closing wedge osteotomy; it is more controllable than closing wedge osteotomy and it restores the height of the deficient knee. Moreover a lateral closing wedge osteotomy shortens a leg in a Varus knee that is typically already short due to medial collapse. The medial opening wedge proximal tibial osteotomy grants greater valgus correction, allows avoiding dissociation of the fibula from the tibia and minimizes or eliminates complications that affect peroneal nerve. Medial opening wedge osteotomy facilitates the treatment of a varus knees with ligament deficiencies [23]. As a matter of fact this method has the possibility to be associated with anterior cruciate ligament reconstruction through the use of the same incision that allows the surgeon to withdraw hamstring tendons and to create the tibial tunnel. Some authors recommend valgus high tibial osteotomy after anterior cruciate ligament reconstruction in Varus knee in order to improve ligament stability and functional results [24]. In the literature we identified two clear indications to perform valgus high tibial osteotomy in patients affected by anterior cruciate ligament deficient knees. The first indication is Varus thrust in double or triple Varus knee and the second indication is represented by medial compartment osteoarthritis in primary Varus knee [25, 26].

Moreover it is possible to perform a chondral resurfacing procedure in conjunction with a high tibial osteotomy in the Varus knee. Resurfacing the degenerative knee will improve results obtained with an osteotomy alone [27].

Surgical Technique for Lateral Opening Wedge Distal Femoral Osteotomy

The patient is placed supine with the knee flexed to 30° using laterally placed side support. Preoperative antibiotics are administered. The incision is on the lateral aspect of the distal third of the femur starting distal to the lateral epicondyle. The skin incision is longitudinal about 12 cm in length. A dissection of the vastus lateral is performed and the muscle is retracted from the postero-lateral intramuscular septum. Two Homan retractors are inserted in order to move the suprapatellar pouch anteriorly and to avoid damage of the posterior vessels posteriorly. With the knee in extension a guide wire is inserted under fluoroscopic control from the lateral aspect of the femur directed to a point few millimeters proximal to the medial epicondyle. The osteotomy is started with an oscillating saw (placed parallel to the guide pin) and is completed with thin osteotomy to increase accuracy and to avoid breakage of the medial cortex. Anterior and posterior cortical bone must be interrupted and at least 1 cm of the medial bone hinge is preserved. Osteotomy must be checked by fluoroscope to grant the appropriate depth and direction of the cut. Slight varus stress is applied using osteotomies until a satisfactory correction is achieved. At which point a "T-shaped" seven holes plate (Puddu plate) was positioned to achieve fixation. 4.5-cortical screws are placed through the holes. A wedge shaped bone graft (allograft) is used to fill the gap. The osteotomy must be perpendicular to the longitudinal axis of the femur in order to hold the plate completely in contact with the lateral femoral cortex (Fig. **4**). *The plate of a lateral opening wedge osteotomy can cause pain by rubbing under the iliotibial band and moreover the osteotomy requires more time for the bone to heal due to the use of bone grafting. It has a higher nonunion rate when comparing to a medial closing wedge osteotomy.*

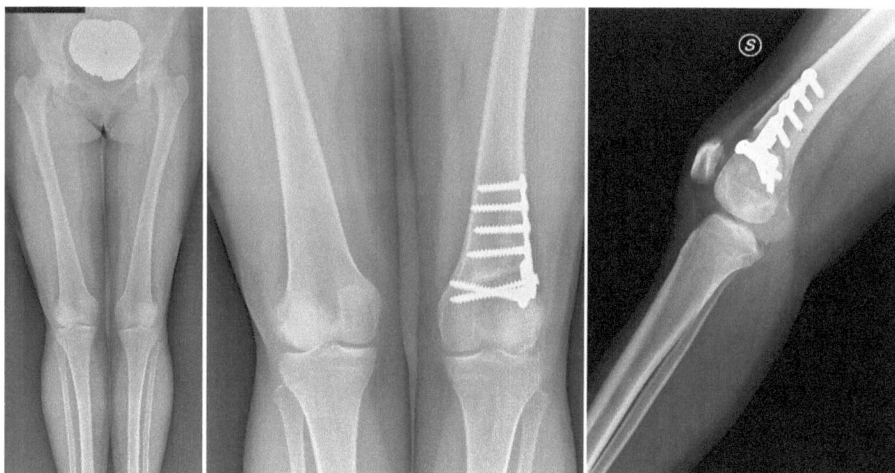

Fig. (4). Preoperative X-rays and postoperative X-rays (A-P view and L-L view) after lateral opening wedge distal femoral osteotomy.

Medial closing wedge distal femoral osteotomy is a well-established procedure for the treatment of the valgus knee. At the moment there is only a locking plate design for the medial side of the distal femur that is the Depuy-Synthes Tomofix medial distal femoral plate. The disadvantages of this surgical procedure are the possible shortening of the lower limb and the higher rate of neurovascular injuries than lateral opening wedge osteotomy.

Postoperative Rehabilitation

The knee is immobilized with a hinged brace in full extension. Patients start rehabilitation program on the first post-operative day with continuous passive motion device, with adjustments of the range of movement from 0° to 60°. The initial pain control is obtained with patient-controlled analgesia by epidural catheter or by parental administration. The limit of the range of movement of the machine of continuous passive motion progressively increases by 10° or more per day according to the tolerance of the patient. The drain is usually removed 24 hours postoperatively. Most patients can be discharged in the second or third postoperative day with a hinged brace applied to the affected leg. This brace allows the patient to perform exercises in order to recover the degree of flexion. Patients are usually able to fully flex the knee within the first four weeks after the surgery. Moreover patients can perform isometric exercises to strengthen the muscles of the leg.

Patients are non-weight bearing until the seven-eight postoperative week and they use crutches for walking. After this period the patients can start a progressive-partial weight bearing. Walking with full weight bearing without assistance is typically achieved at third postoperative month if there is radiographic evidence that the bone has sufficiently healed. Excessive early joint loading and premature excessive knee flexion-extension with external loads can compromise bone healing and the integrity of the surgical realignment.

Complications

Correct patient selection is mandatory to minimize major complications. Knowledge of the history of the patient, physical examination, radiographic assessment with full-lengths standing films planned preoperatively and arthroscopic evaluation performed before osteotomy are all procedures that might be observed to avoid complications.

In HTO we try to keep the knee at 90° of flexion in order to avoid neurovascular bundle iatrogenic injuries. We usually start the osteotomy with electric saw blade and we ultimate the procedure with a hand-osteotomy tool to clearly check the limit of the cut (10 mm of the far cortex must be preserved). In HTO the tibial plateau must be at least 10 mm thick to avoid fracture. Fluoroscopy must be constantly used to evaluate the deepening of the cut and the eventual iatrogenic misalignment.

If a fracture occurs an internal fixation can be performed. The possible post-surgical procedure complications of osteotomy are [2]: -under correction, overcorrection and loss of correction, restricted range of motion, intra-articular fracture, nonunion, infection, patella baja, compartment syndrome, peroneal nerve dysfunction, and osteonecrosis of the proximal fragment, vascular injury and thromboembolic disease. A fracture can be treated with internal fixation while patella baja can be corrected with a revision procedure or by a total knee arthroplasty.

CONFLICT OF INTEREST

The authors confirm that the author have no conflict of interest to declare for this publication.

ACKNOWLEDGEMENTS

We would like to thank Luigi Lena (Rizzoli Orthopaedic Institute) for his help with the images.

REFERENCES

[1]   Amis A. Biomechanics of high tibial osteotomy. Knee surgery, sports traumatology, arthroscopy: official. Journal of the ESSKA 2013; 21: 197-205.
       [http://dx.doi.org/10.1007/s00167-012-2122-3]

[2]   Insall JN, Scott WN. Surgery of the knee. Third. Churchill Livingstone, editor. 2000.

[3]   Foroughi N, Smith R, Vanwanseele B. The association of external knee adduction moment with biomechanical variables in osteoarthritis: a systematic review. Knee 2009; 16(5): 303-9.
       [http://dx.doi.org/10.1016/j.knee.2008.12.007] [PMID: 19321348]

[4]   Andriacchi TP, Mündermann A, Smith RL, Alexander EJ, Dyrby CO, Koo S. A framework for the *in vivo* pathomechanics of osteoarthritis at the knee. Ann Biomed Eng 2004; 32(3): 447-57.
       [http://dx.doi.org/10.1023/B:ABME.0000017541.82498.37] [PMID: 15095819]

[5]   Lind M, McClelland J, Wittwer JE, Whitehead TS, Feller JA, Webster KE. Gait analysis of walking before and after medial opening wedge high tibial osteotomy. Knee Surg Sports Traumatol Arthrosc 2013; 21(1): 74-81.
       [http://dx.doi.org/10.1007/s00167-011-1496-y] [PMID: 21484389]

[6]   McMahon M, Block JA. The risk of contralateral total knee arthroplasty after knee replacement for osteoarthritis. J Rheumatol 2003; 30(8): 1822-4.
       [PMID: 12913941]

[7]   Lobenhoffer P, Agneskirchner JD. Improvements in surgical technique of valgus high tibial osteotomy. Knee surgery, sports traumatology, arthroscopy. official journal of the ESSKA 2003; 11: 132-8.

[8]   Staubli AE, De Simoni C, Babst R, Lobenhoffer P. TomoFix: a new LCP-concept for open wedge osteotomy of the medial proximal tibia early results in 92 cases. Injury 2003; 34 (Suppl. 2): B55-62.
       [http://dx.doi.org/10.1016/j.injury.2003.09.025] [PMID: 14580986]

[9]   Virolainen P, Aro HT. High tibial osteotomy for the treatment of osteoarthritis of the knee: a review of the literature and a meta-analysis of follow-up studies. Arch Orthop Trauma Surg 2004; 124(4): 258-61.
         [http://dx.doi.org/10.1007/s00402-003-0545-5] [PMID: 12827394]

[10]   Amendola A, Panarella L. High tibial osteotomy for the treatment of unicompartmental arthritis of the knee. Orthop Clin North Am 2005; 36(4): 497-504.
         [http://dx.doi.org/10.1016/j.ocl.2005.05.009] [PMID: 16164954]

[11]   Naudie D, Bourne RB, Rorabeck CH, Bourne TJ. The Install Award. Survivorship of the high tibial valgus osteotomy. A 10- to -22-year followup study. Clin Orthop Relat Res 1999; (367): 18-27.
         [PMID: 10546594]

[12]   Flecher X, Parratte S, Aubaniac J-M, Argenson J-N. A 1228-year followup study of closing wedge high tibial osteotomy. Clin Orthop Relat Res 2006; 452(452): 91-6.
         [http://dx.doi.org/10.1097/01.blo.0000229362.12244.f6] [PMID: 16906111]

[13]   Aglietti P, Rinonapoli E, Stringa G, Taviani A. Tibial osteotomy for the Varus osteoarthritic knee. Clin Orthop Relat Res 1983; (176): 239-51. 1983/06/01 ed

[14]   Surin V, Markhede G, Sundholm K. Factors influencing results of high tibial osteotomy in gonarthrosis. Acta Orthop Scand 1975; 46(6): 996-1007.
         [http://dx.doi.org/10.3109/17453677508989289] [PMID: 1211137]

[15]   Tigani D, Ferrari D, Trentani P, Barbanti-Brodano G, Trentani F. Patellar height after high tibial osteotomy. Int Orthop 2001; 24(6): 331-4.
         [http://dx.doi.org/10.1007/s002640000173] [PMID: 11294424]

[16]   Stukenborg-Colsman C, Wirth CJ, Lazovic D, Wefer A. High tibial osteotomy *versus* unicompartmental joint replacement in unicompartmental knee joint osteoarthritis: 7-10-year follow-up prospective randomized study. Knee 2001; 8(3): 187-94. 2001/11/15 ed.

[17]   Bonnin M, Amendola A, Bellemans J, MacDonald S, Ménétrey J. The Knee Joint. Paris: Springer Paris 2012, pp. 633-41.
         [http://dx.doi.org/10.1007/978-2-287-99353-4]

[18]   Dettoni F, Bonasia DE, Castoldi F, Bruzzone M, Blonna D, Rossi R. High tibial osteotomy *versus* unicompartmental knee arthroplasty for medial compartment arthrosis of the knee: a review of the literature. Iowa Orthop J 2010; 30: 131-40.
         [PMID: 21045985]

[19]   Coventry MB, Ilstrup DM, Wallrichs SL. Proximal tibial osteotomy. A critical long-term study of eighty-seven cases. J Bone Joint Surg Am 1993; 75(2): 196-201.
         [PMID: 8423180]

[20]   Job-Deslandre C, Languepin A, Benvenuto M, Menkès CJ. Tibial valgization osteotomy in gonarthrosis with or without chondrocalcinosis. Results after 5 years. Revue du rhumatisme et des maladies ostéo-articulaires ; 58(7): 491-6.

[21]   Bauer GC, Insall J, Koshino T. Tibial osteotomy in gonarthrosis (osteo-arthritis of the knee). J Bone Joint Surg Am 1969; 51(8): 1545-63.
         [PMID: 5357176]

[22]   Gaasbeek RD, Toonen HG, van Heerwaarden RJ, Buma P. Mechanism of bone incorporation of beta-TCP bone substitute in open wedge tibial osteotomy in patients. Biomaterials 2005; 26(33): 6713-9.
[http://dx.doi.org/10.1016/j.biomaterials.2005.04.056] [PMID: 15950278]

[23]   Seagrave RA, Sojka J, Goodyear A, Munns SW. Utilizing reamer irrigator aspirator (RIA) autograft for opening wedge high tibial osteotomy: A new surgical technique and report of three cases. Int J Surg Case Rep 2014; 5(1): 37-42.
[http://dx.doi.org/10.1016/j.ijscr.2013.11.004] [PMID: 24412805]

[24]   Kim S-J, Moon H-K, Chun Y-M, Chang W-H, Kim S-G. Is correctional osteotomy crucial in primary varus knees undergoing anterior cruciate ligament reconstruction? Clin Orthop Relat Res 2011; 469(5): 1421-6.
[http://dx.doi.org/10.1007/s11999-010-1584-1] [PMID: 20872103]

[25]   Badhe NP, Forster IW. High tibial osteotomy in knee instability: the rationale of treatment and early results. Knee surg sport traumatol arthroscopy 2002; 10: 38-43.
[http://dx.doi.org/10.1007/s001670100244]

[26]   Lattermann C, Jakob RP. High tibial osteotomy alone or combined with ligament reconstruction in anterior cruciate ligament-deficient knees. Knee surg sport traumatol arthroscopy 1996; 4: 32-8.
[http://dx.doi.org/10.1007/BF01565995]

[27]   Sterett WI, Steadman JR. Chondral resurfacing and high tibial osteotomy in the Varus knee. Am J Sport Med 2004; 32(5): 1243-49.
[http://dx.doi.org/10.1177/0363546503259301]

CHAPTER 8

Total Knee Replacement in Arthritis - Current Concepts

Narayan Hulse[*]

Fortis Hospital, Banneragatta Road, Bengaluru, India

Abstract: Total knee replacement is one of the most successful and cost-effective interventions in the modern medicine for the treatment of pain caused by advanced arthritis of the knee. Great advances have been made in the last five decades in the mechanical properties and the design of the knee implants, surgical techniques and prevention of complications. Both cruciate-retaining and sacrificing designs are widely used with the proponents of both the designs. More constrained designs are used in complex primary and in revision cases. Pain affecting the activities of daily living in an elderly person suffering from severe osteoarthritis is the commonest indication for a primary total knee arthroplasty followed by rheumatoid arthritis. Current or recent infection is an absolute contraindication for a knee replacement. Most commonly the procedure is performed through a midline longitudinal incision and a medial parapatellar arthrotomy. Recent advances include computer aided navigation (has shown to improve the component positioning), gender specific knee (better choice of component sizes) and patient specific instrumentation (to improve the accuracy of bone resection). Long term results and cost effectiveness of these techniques remain unproven. Infection (1-3%) is the most common and serious complication followed by thromboembolism, instability, and neurovascular injury.

Keywords: Knee implants, Osteoarthritis, Primary knee replacement, Revision knee arthroplasty, Rheumatoid arthritis, Surgical treatment of arthritis, Total knee arthroplasty, Total knee designs, Total knee replacement.

---

[*] **Corresponding author Narayan Hulse:** Fortis Hospital, Bannergatta Road, Bengaluru, India, 560076; Tel; +91 9591382501; E-mail: drnhulse@gmail.com

Ashish Anand (Ed.)

INTRODUCTION

Total knee arthroplasty is one of the most successful and cost-effective interventions for the treatment of severe arthritis (Fig. **1**) of the knee [1]. Number of procedures performed each year have been increased tremendously in the last decade and it has been projected to increase further in the coming years [2, 3]. Many studies have documented over 95% of survival of these components, over 15 years of follow-up [4 - 6].

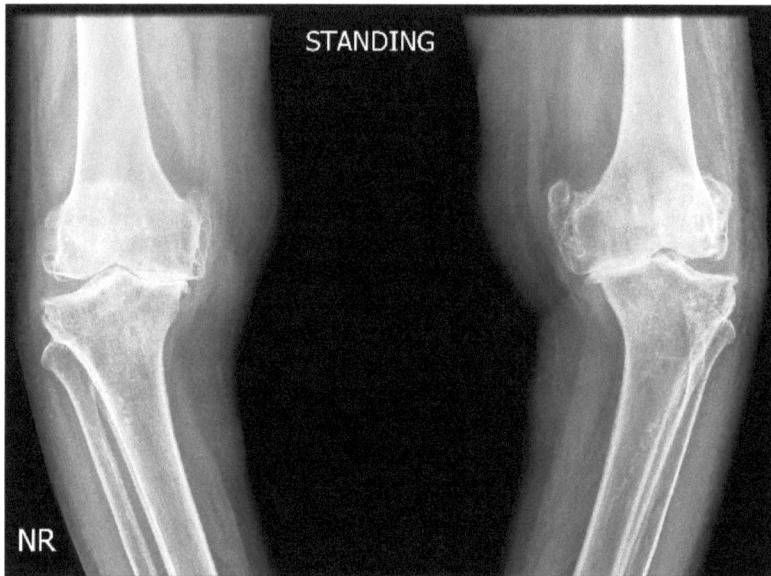

Fig. (1). Severe osteoarthritis of the knee.

COMPONENT DESIGN AND HISTORICAL PERSPECTIVE

Interposition of metallic components in the knee to relieve pain began with the work of Campbell (distal femoral metallic mould) [7], Macintosh (tibia mould) [8], and McKeever (tibial tray with a keel) [9]. This was followed by the development of hinged designs like Walldius hinge [10] and Guepar hinge [11]. Total condylar prosthesis designed by Insall and others in 1973 ushered the modern era of total knee arthroplasty [12]. This design improved many previous prostheses in terms of stability and survivorship. In this design both the cruciate ligaments were sacrificed. Stability was attained by the congruity of the articular surfaces.

Antero-posterior translation of the components were resisted by the anterior and posterior lips of the tibial component and the median eminence. Double dish design of the tibial polyethylene component provided stability in extension and coronal plane stability in flexion. Femoral component was made from cobalt chrome alloy whereas all poly tibial component was later changed to metal back. Patellar polyethylene dome had single peg for fixation. To prevent the posterior dislocation reported in the total condylar design, the Insall-Burstein posterior cruciate-substituting or posterior-stabilized design was developed in 1978 by adding a central cam mechanism to the articular surface geometry of the total condylar prosthesis [13].

Another milestone was the development of kinematic knee prosthesis which was evolved from duo patellar prosthesis where PCL retention was possible [14]. Originally medial and lateral tibial components were separate, but later on these components were joined to make a single tibial component. This design was widely used in 1980s. Patellar complications were significantly high in 1980*s* and 1990s [15]. Most of the current designs are derivatives of the Insall-Burstein and kinematic designs. Newer designs incorporate greater areas of patello-femoral contact through a larger range of motion and asymmetrical anterior flanges designed to resist patellar subluxation.

COMPONENT DESIGN AND CHOICE OF IMPLANTS

Choice of components of a modern total knee arthroplasty depends on the available bone stock, integrity of the cruciate ligaments and collateral ligaments. Increasing degree of constraint is incorporated in the various designs to compensate for the deficiencies in these structures.

Cruciate Retaining Knee (CR)

Cruciate retaining knee designs incorporate the least amount of constraint among the various designs of the total knee components (Fig. **2**). This design allows retaining the posterior cruciate ligament. Theoretical advantages include, better roll back and more natural gait especially while climbing the stairs, bone preservation and less strain on the metal-bone interface [16, 17]. However these claims are difficult to establish in the clinical studies. Reported disadvantages include, difficulty in balancing the flexion space and in a chronically arthritic knee PCL may not be functional or may be incompetent especially in rheumatoid arthritis.

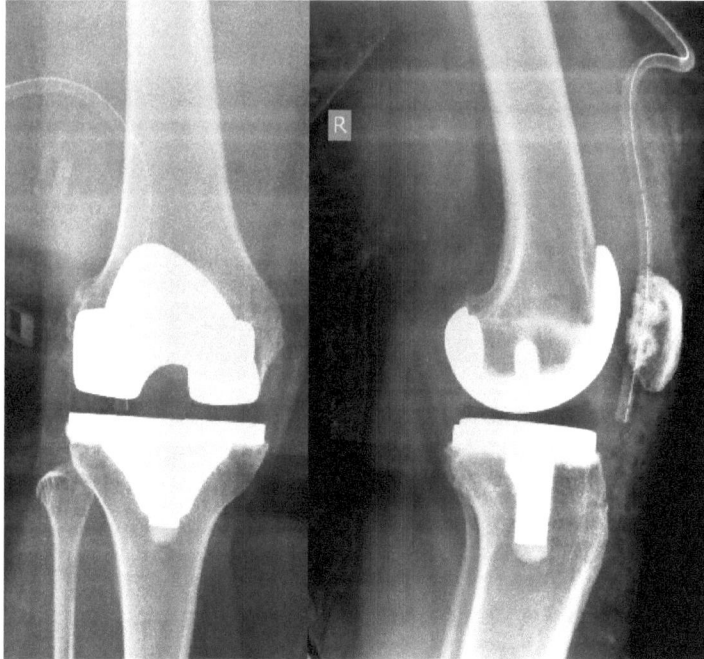

Fig. (2). Cruciate retaining knee prosthesis in place.

Posterior Stabilized Knee (PS)

Cruciate substituting or posterior stabilized knees have a post and cam mechanism to prevent posterior translation of tibia in flexion [13]. Currently this is one of the most commonly used designs. These designs need resection of the intercondylar notch to accommodate the cam and post mechanism. Indications for PCL retaining and cruciate substituting designs are still controversial. Multiple studies have found no significant differences in the function, patient satisfaction or survivorship between these two designs [18 - 21].

Mobile Bearing Prostheses

To reduce the stress at bone-prosthesis interface, mobile bearing knees were introduced. Some degree of mobility was incorporated between the polyethylene insert and the tibial component [22, 23]. In the LCS (Low contact stress knee), Buechel and others incorporated many of the features of the earlier Oxford knee [24, 25]. Individual polyethylene menisci articulated with the femoral component above and with a polished tibial baseplate below. Jordan, Olivo and Voorhorst reported a survival rate of 94% for the cementless version of this design after 8 years of follow up [26]. Buechel, one of the developers of the LCS design, reported a 98%, 20-year survivorship with this design and a similar survivorship at 18 years with the cementless rotating platform design [24]. This design had rare rotational dislocations of the tibial inserts if the flexion and extension gap was not balanced adequately during surgery [25, 26]. Potential advantages of mobile bearing knees include lower contact stresses at the articulating surfaces, rotational motion of the tibial polyethylene during gait and self-alignment of the tibial polyethylene compensating for small rotational malalignment of the tibial baseplate during implantation [22 - 26].

Varus-Valgus Constrained Knee

The original constrained condylar knee (CCK) was developed by Insall and others from the posterior-substituting designs [27]. Varus-valgus constrained implants (Fig. **3**) were designed to provide stability in coronal plate to compensate for the collateral ligament deficiencies. These implants have a tall tibial post which engages in a deep femoral box providing inherent stability. These implants are used commonly in revisions and complex primary procedures with ligament deficiencies. These constrained implants impart greater stress at the implant-bone interface and hence they are commonly used along with stem extenders to improve the stability of the fixation. These implants may be used for both primary and revision arthroplasty, particularly for severe valgus deformity, collateral ligament deficiency, bone defects, and residual instability or uncorrectable flexion-extension imbalances. Rosenberg, Verner, and Galante reported progressive radiolucencies in 16% of patients at an average of 44 months after using the total condylar prosthesis III, the precursor of the CCK [28]. Donaldson *et al.* reported no failures at 4-year follow-up in 17 primary arthroplasties with the total condylar prosthesis III in knees with severe valgus deformities; five failures occurred in 14 revision arthroplasties [29]. Most total knee systems include a variation of the varus-valgus constrained design.

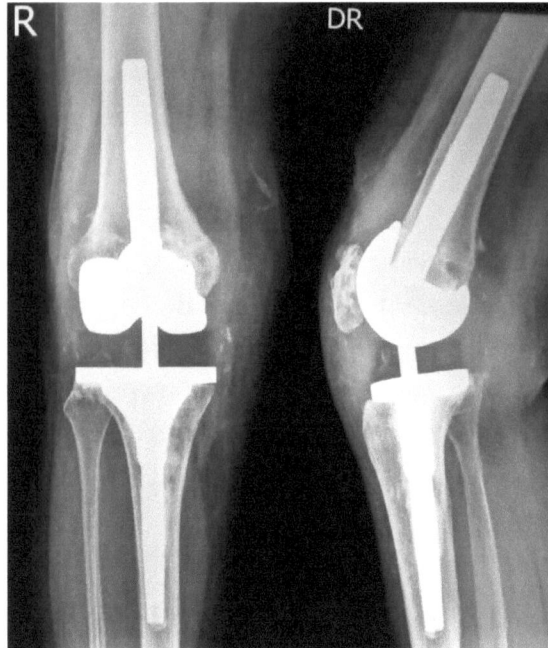

Fig. (3). Varus valgus Constrained Implant.

Rotating-Hinge Knee

Rotating hinge implants (Fig. **4**) are designed for complex revisions with severe instability, bone loss and for skeletal malignancies. They are highly constrained devices and hence used in extreme situations only. Hinges restrict coronal plane and translational forces. This prosthesis also allows the knee to rotate approximately by 10°, reproducing normal kinematics. The femoral and tibial components are secured to the bone by intramedullary stems [30].

Originally hinged prosthesis was developed for massive knee reconstruction after tumour resections [31]. These fixed hinge designs allowed movement of only one axis of flexion and extension only. This lead to excessive stress on the prosthesis bone interface leading to early aseptic loosening. This lead to the introduction of rotating hinge designs [30, 32]. Later modular fluted stems, medullary cones were also introduced. Because of higher incidence of complications and shorter survival rates, these components are reserved for elderly patients with limited mobility [32 - 34].

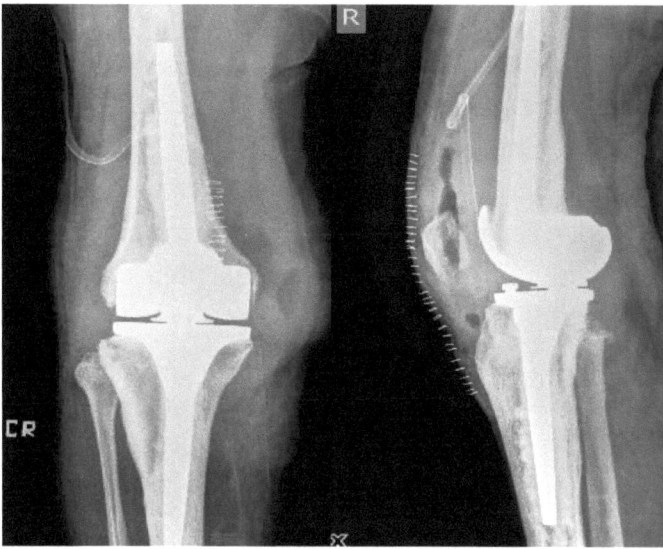

Fig. (4). Rotating hinge knee replacement following a revision for infection.

High Flexion Knee

Demand for higher flexion after total knee arthroplasty and the cultural need for higher flexion in some parts of the word, lead to the concept of high-flexion knees. Usually patients who underwent total knee arthroplasty achieve about 110° of flexion on average. Amount of flexion in the knee depends on multiple factors like preoperative flexion, body weight and various component designs. Most consistent predictor of postoperative flexion is range of preoperative flexion [34 - 36].

Modifications in the design of total knee arthroplasty to achieve higher flexion include lengthening the radius of curvature through the posterior condyles, increasing the posterior condylar offset, recessing the tibial insert, lengthening the trochlear groove, and altering the cam-post design [34]. These changes allow increased femoral rollback, translation, and thus, clearance in deep flexion. Several high-flexion prostheses are now available and show variable results. None of the high-flexion designs so far shown statistically significant improvement in the flexion compared to standard prosthesis [35, 36].

Gender-Specific Knee

Surgeons have always faced a situation of disparity between the sizes of male and female knees especially the medio-lateral dimension of the distal femur compared to corresponding anteroposterior dimension [37 - 39]. Gender specific knee components to accommodate the anatomic differences between men and women have been developed. Theoretical benefit of decreasing the medio-lateral overhang of the femoral components in women should result in better clinical outcome is controversial [39 - 41]. Thomsen *et al.* showed significant improvements in several gait parameters after the knee arthroplasty without evidence of any significant advantages attributable to the gender-specific design [39].

INDICATION FOR TOTAL KNEE ARTHROPLASTY

1. Primary indication is to relieve knee pain from severe arthritis in elderly patients (Fig. **1**). TKA is indicated when conservative methods found inadequate to relieve pain and improve function satisfactorily. Common factors to consider include, difficulty with the activities of daily living, frequent analgesic usage and night pain [40].
2. Most commonly performed for osteoarthritis followed by rheumatoid arthritis. However, TKA is also performed in variety of arthritic conditions when medical management fails to control pain. For example, Psoriatic arthritis, post traumatic or secondary osteoarthritis, osteochondromatosis, pseudogout, chondocalcinosis *etc.*
3. Survival of a knee replacement in an individual patient may be shorter than the survival of a patient. Hence this procedure is indicated preferably in elderly patients. However, in systemic arthritis and similar conditions this procedure may be performed in younger individuals to improve their mobility and function.
4. Total knee arthroplasty is occasionally indicated for severe knee deformities in elderly, *e.g.* sever flexion deformity, varus-valgus instability *etc.*

CONTRAINDICATIONS

1. Absolute contraindications include recent or current knee sepsis, a remote

source of ongoing infection, extensor mechanism discontinuity or severe extensor dysfunction, recurvatum deformity secondary to muscular weakness and the presence of a painless, well-functioning knee arthrodesis [42].

2. Relative contraindications are numerous and debatable and include medical conditions that compromise the patient's ability to withstand anaesthesia, the metabolic demands of surgery and wound healing, and the significant rehabilitation necessary to ensure a favourable functional outcome.

3. Other relative contraindications include significant atherosclerotic disease of the operative leg, skin conditions such as psoriasis within the operative field, venous stasis disease with recurrent cellulitis, neuropathic arthropathy, morbid obesity, recurrent urinary tract infections and a history of osteomyelitis in the proximity of the knee.

SURGICAL TECHNIQUES

Surgical Approach

Patient is positioned supine with the knee flexed to 90° using a foot support and a thigh support attached the operating table. Most of the surgery is performed with the knee in flexion to displace the popliteal neurovascular structures posteriorly, away from the surgical field. Anterior longitudinal midline and medial parapatellar retinacular incision is most commonly used. In case of a single previous scar, same can be used if it is in a usable location or that can be incorporated into the new incision. A healthy skin bridge of about 7cm is recommended if a new parallel longitudinal incision is needed. In case of multiple previous scars, most lateral scar should be used. Previous transverse scars which were historically used for various surgical procedures like open reduction of patella should be ignored [42].

Other approaches are subvastus, midvastus and lateral approaches. The subvastus approach was described by Hofmann, Plaster and Murdock. This approach leaves the extensor mechanism intact. Potential benefits include rapid return of quadriceps strength, preservation of the vascularity to patella, improved patient satisfaction while decreasing the postoperative pain and lesser need for lateral release [43, 44]. However, extent of the exposure may be limited especially in obese patients and patients with previous knee surgeries [43, 44].

Engh and Parks described the midvastus approach, which differs from the subvastus approach in that the vastus medialis muscle is split in line with its fibres, rather than subluxated laterally in its entirety [45]. The split in the vastus medialis muscle starts at the superomedial border of the patella and extends proximally and medially toward the intermuscular septum. This approach preserves the superior genicular artery to the patella and the quadriceps tendon. Relative contraindications to the midvastus approach include obesity, previous high tibial osteotomy and preoperative flexion of less than 80 degrees [45, 46].

Lateral approach is used by some authors for valgus knees [47]. Theoretical benefit includes, easy access to lateral structures where major soft tissue release may be required to correct the valgus deformity. However, majority of the surgeons use more familiar medial parapatellar approach even for the valgus knees without much difficulty.

Mini-Incision Techniques

Different techniques and instruments have been developed to reduce the length of the surgical scar [48]. Other than the smaller surgical scar, theoretical advantages include, quadriceps sparing, lesser blood loss and early rehabilitation. These approaches are technically demanding and risks higher complication rates. Smaller length of the surgical incision is facilitated by use of smaller specialised instruments, avoiding patellar eversion, *in situ* bone resection without dislocating the knee [48].

Bone Preparation

Preparation of the bone to seat the components is done using mechanical jigs provided by the specific implant manufacturers. Surgical steps of the procedure vary depending on the make of the component and the preference of the operating surgeon. However general guiding principles remain same for most of the modern implants. Following important principles are followed. A) Restoring the mechanical axis of the lower limb, B) Restoring the normal rotation of the femoral and tibial components, C) Sizing components to prevent overstuffing, and loose gaps or overhanging of components D) Obtaining equal flexion and extension gaps E) thumb free patellar tracking [42].

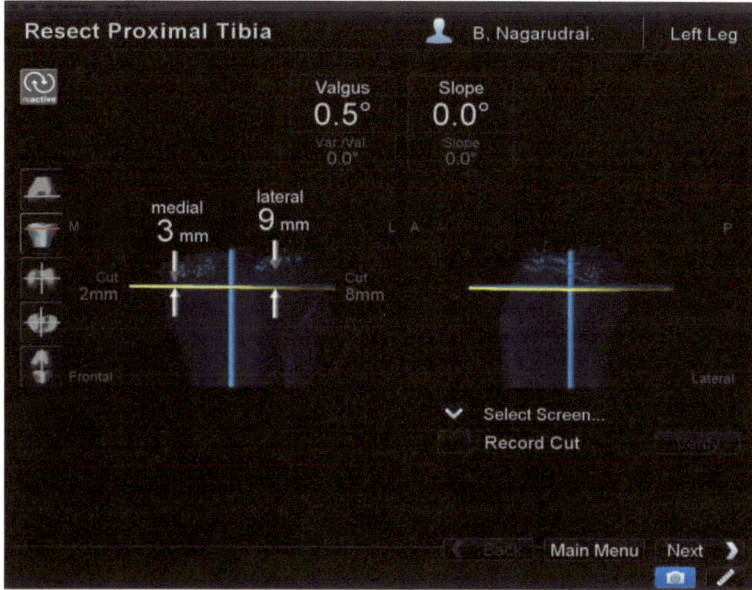

Fig. (5). Output as seen in the monitor during a computer navigation.

Computer-Assisted Techniques

Coronal plane mal-alignment of more than 3° has been shown to increase the aseptic loosening of the implants [49]. Various computerised devices to assist the bone preparation during a total knee arthroplasty have been developed in the last decade. Navigation machines could be imageless systems which need no preoperative imaging, whereas others are image based systems which utilise preoperative CT scans or fluoroscopy images [50, 51]. Computer (Fig. **5**) records the orientation of multiple bony landmarks with the help of variety of sensors [50]. Using these bony landmarks which are recorded during the registration process, mechanical and anatomical axes, rotational and sagittal alignment and the size of the components are determined. Regardless of the technique used, improved alignment has been documented by multiple authors compared to conventional methods [51]. Although complications attributable to the computer-assisted technique have been infrequent, increased operative time and increased cost have limited its widespread acceptance. Long-term studies are needed to assess the improved outcome as a result of more reproducible implant positioning [51 - 54].

Patient Specific Instrumentation (PSI)

Patient-specific instrumentation (Fig. **6**) involves recording of patient's bony landmarks preoperatively and creation of digital image and creation of customised cutting blocks preoperatively, whereas registration process of most of the navigation system happens during surgery [55]. All these systems require preoperative MRI or CT, with specifications determined by the instrument manufacturer [55, 56]. Claimed advantages of PSI incudes greater accuracy in coronal alignment with fewer outliers, no violation of intramedullary canal of femur and tibia, lesser surgical time, lower hospital costs and improved clinical outcomes [55, 56]. Few published studies failed to conclusively prove the advantages and clinical outcomes [56, 57, 59]. Disadvantages include increased cost of imaging and manufacturing the custom instruments as well as increased preoperative time required from the day of imaging to manufacturing the custom jigs [57 - 59]. As in the navigation systems, a standard set of instrumentation is also needed to be available in the operation theatre.

Decisive evidence exists to support the fact that PSI requires fewer surgical trays. PSI has neither clearly been shown to improve the surgical efficiency nor the cost-effectiveness of TKA. Mid and long-term data regarding PSI's effect on functional outcomes and component survivorship do not exist and short-term data are scarce. When PSI is compared with the traditional instrumentation, available literature does not clearly show better in terms of postoperative pain, activity, function and range of motion [57 - 59].

Resurfacing *versus* Not Resurfacing Patella

This is one of the long drawn controversies in TKA [60]. Successful outcomes supporting both resurfacing and non-resurfacing patella are available in the literature [61 - 63]. Proponents of patellar resurfacing claim less anterior knee pain and less reoperation rate after patellar resurfacing. Patellar complications were higher in the earlier designs because of unfriendly trochlear grove of the femoral component. Complications of patella resurfacing include patella fracture, loosening of the component, peg failure and overstuffing [60].

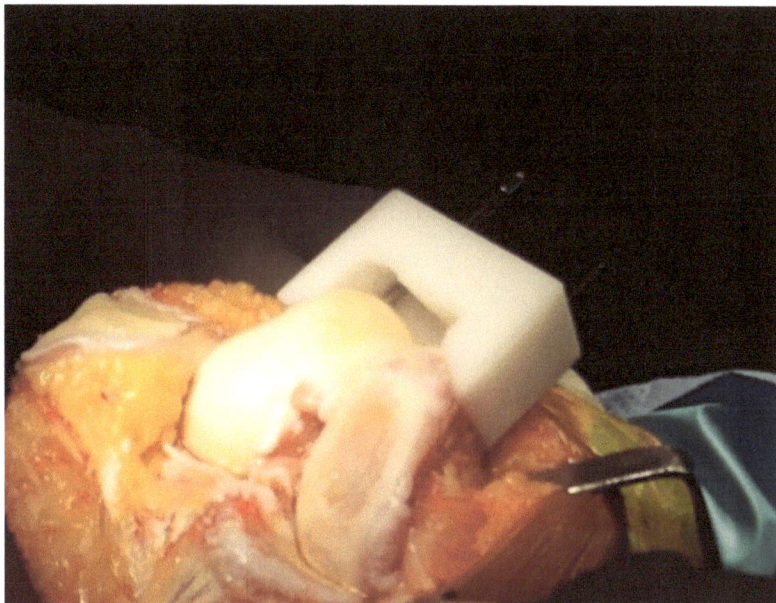

Fig. (6). Customise Instruments (Patient specific instrumentation).

Cemented *vs* Cementless Fixation

While cemented fixation is considered as a gold standard, researchers have attempted uncemented fixation also. Implants with various coatings and ingrowth surfaces have been developed for uncemented implantation [63, 64]. Cementless fixation has not shown a similar success in TKA that has been seen in total hip arthroplasty, despite many attempts to perfect this technique [63 - 65].

COMPLICATIONS

Infection

Rate of Infection (Fig. **7**) after knee arthroplasties ranges from 1% to-3%. Acceptable modern standard is about 1% [42, 66 - 68]. Single dose of intravenous antibiotic at the time of anaesthetic induction, modern aseptic surgical techniques, laminar flow operation theatres, antibiotic impregnated cement and body exhaust suites have contributed immensely for reduction of infection. Acute infection may be salvaged with a thorough debridement and polyethylene exchange. However severe infection with implant loosening usually requires two stage revision arthroplasty [66 - 68].

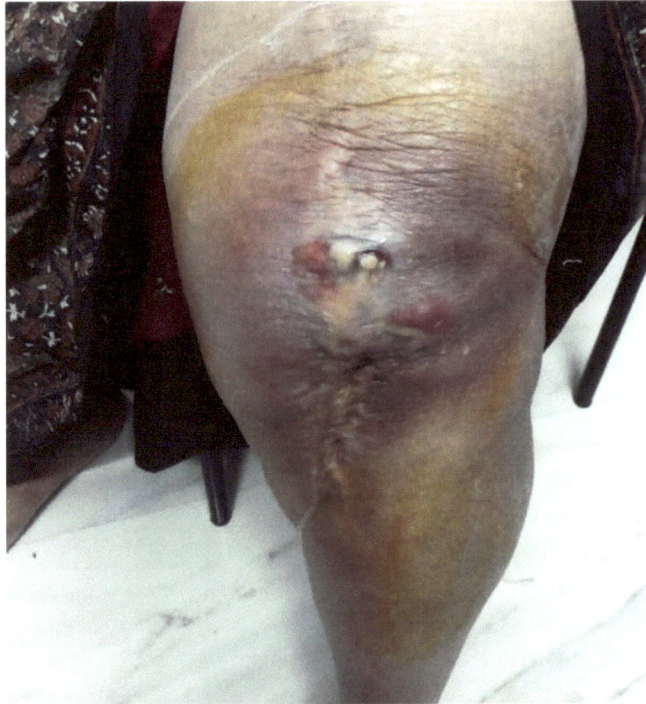

Fig. (7). Infected total knee with abscess.

Instability

Instability is one of the common complications of total knee arthroplasty, which accounts for about 10-20% of revisions [66, 67, 69]. Symptomatic instability occurs in about 1-2% of patients. Instability occurs both in coronal and sagittal plane. Both technical and patient factors contribute for instability *e.g.* improper balancing of collateral ligaments, unequal flexion and extension gaps, mal-positioning of components, bone loss or over resection, late loosening and connective tissue laxity. Treatment depends on the severity and the cause of instability. Minor instability could be managed with bracing and physiotherapy, whereas major instability may need poly exchange, revision or a constrained device [68 - 70].

Vascular Injury

Popliteal artery injury during saw cuts or dissection is an uncommon but a catastrophic complication. In 90° flexion of the knee, popliteal artery is about 9 mm behind the posterior cortex of tibia [42]. If arterial injury is suspected, the tourniquet must be deflated to check for arterial bleeding, distal pulses or a hand held intraoperative Doppler. Arterial repair with the help of a vascular surgeon is usually required as an emergency procedure [42, 69, 70].

Nerve Palsy

Common peroneal nerve injury resulting in foot drop is rare but could occur after correction of severe valgus and flexion deformities. If suspected knee should be kept in flexion during pot operative period to reduce tension. Initial treatment incudes splints and physical therapy [42, 68, 69].

Wound Complications

Wound dehiscence and other wound complications are rare but seen in immunocompromised patients, correction of complex deformities and previous extensive scaring on the knee (Fig. **8**) [42, 68 - 70].

Deep Vein Thrombosis (DVT) and Pulmonary Embolism (PE)

Routine DVT prophylaxis is recommended for all the patients undergoing total knee arthroplasties. Incidence of fatal pulmonary embolism is about 0.001% after TKA [42, 68 - 70].

Stiffness

Stiffness could result due to various factors like pre-operative stiff knees, obesity, inadequate physiotherapy and intra operative technical faults. If patient achieves less than 90° of flexion at 6 to 8 weeks, manipulation under anaesthesia is attempted if the components are satisfactorily [42, 68 - 71].

Other Complications

Regional pain syndrome, patellar complications, anterior knee pain and periprosthetic fractures [42, 68 - 73].

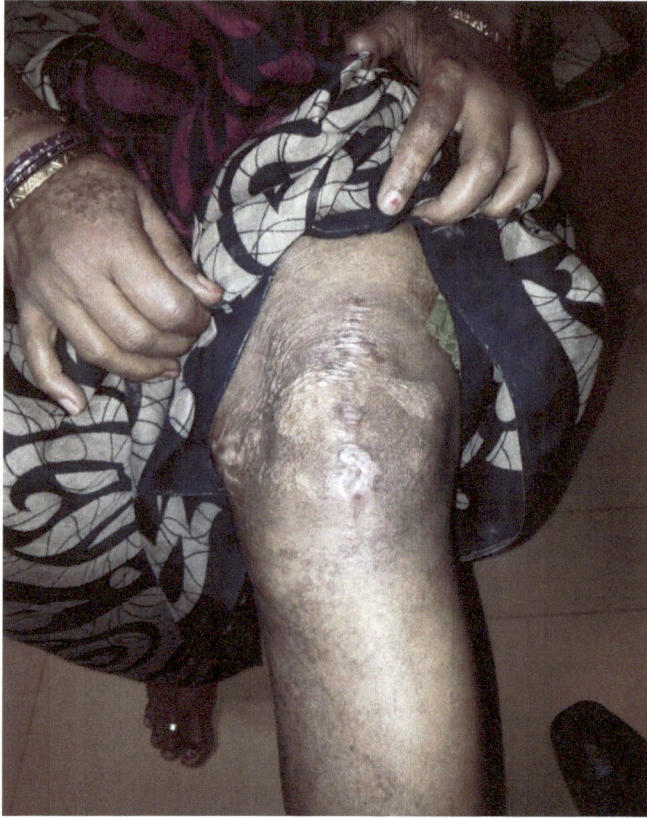

Fig. (8). Prior scar secondary to burns.

UNCOMPARTMENTAL KNEE REPLACEMENTS

Unicompartmental or partial knee replacements were introduced about three decades ago to deal with arthritis involving isolated single compartment of the knee in relatively younger patients. Implants are available for isolated medial, lateral and patellofemoral arthritis. Advantages include lower perioperative morbidity and earlier recovery compared to total knee arthroplasties. Tibial polyethylene inserts are available in fixed and mobile bearing designs. Both designs can yield excellent clinical outcomes at 10 years, but with different modes of long-term failure [74]. Unicompartmental knee offers advantages of lower infection rates, preserving bone stock, minimizing invasiveness and restoring knee kinematics without sacrificing ligaments [75]. However, in many studies, survivorship of UKAs is poorer than that of TKAs especially aseptic loosening [76, 77].

NATIONAL JOINT REGISTRIES

National joint registries collect information related to joint replacement surgery and their outcomes from a large number of patients at national level. These registries provide data for various researches and considered to be one of the most reliable sources of information. Registries could be used as a surveillance tool to monitor the performance of the implants. Scandinavian counties started the oldest joint registries, with over 30 countries now having their own joint registries. Registries are useful for identifying procedure incidence and device utilization, evaluating outcomes, determining patients at risk for complications and reoperations, identifying devices in recall situations, assessing comparative effectiveness of procedures and devices, and providing data for research studies [78].

CONFLICT OF INTEREST

The author confirms that the author has no conflict of interest to declare for this publication.

ACKNOWLEDGEMENTS

Declared none.

REFERENCES

[1] Richmond J, Hunter D, Irrgang J, *et al.* American Academy of Orthopaedic Surgeons clinical practice guideline on the treatment of osteoarthritis (OA) of the knee. J Bone Joint Surg Am 2010; 92(4): 990-3.
[http://dx.doi.org/10.2106/JBJS.I.00982] [PMID: 20360527]

[2] Weinstein AM, Rome BN, Reichmann WM, *et al.* Estimating the burden of total knee replacement in the United States. J Bone Joint Surg Am 2013; 95(5): 385-92.
[http://dx.doi.org/10.2106/JBJS.L.00206] [PMID: 23344005]

[3] Steiner C, Andrews R, Barrett M, Weiss A. HCUP Projections: mobility/orthopaedic procedures 2011 to 2012. HCUP projections report 2012-03.

[4] US Agency for Healthcare Research and Quality website. www.hcup-us.ahrq.gov/reports/projections/2012-03.pdf. Published September 20, 2012. Accessed May 8, 2013.

[5]   Font-Rodriguez DE, Scuderi GR, Insall JN. Survivorship of cemented total knee arthroplasty. Clin Orthop Relat Res 1997; (345): 79-86.
        [PMID: 9418624]

[6]   Ranawat CS, Flynn WF Jr, Saddler S, Hansraj KK, Maynard MJ. Long-term results of the total condylar knee arthroplasty. A 15-year survivorship study. Clin Orthop Relat Res 1993; (286): 94-102.
        [PMID: 8425373]

[7]   Ritter MA, Herbst SA, Keating EM, Faris PM, Meding JB. Long-term survival analysis of a posterior cruciate-retaining total condylar total knee arthroplasty. Clin Orthop Relat Res 1994; (309): 136-45.
        [PMID: 7994952]

[8]   Campbell WC. Interposition of vitallium plates in arthroplasties of the knee: Preliminary report. Am J Surg 1940; 47: 639.
        [http://dx.doi.org/10.1016/S0002-9610(40)90176-3]

[9]   MacIntosh DL. Arthroplasty of the knee in rheumatoid arthritis. J Bone Joint Surg 1966; 48: 179.

[10]   McKeever DC. Tibial plateau prosthesis. Clin Orthop 1960; (18): 86-95.
        [PMID: 16239775]

[11]   Walldius B. Arthroplasty of the knee joint employing an acrylic prosthesis. Acta Orthop Scand 1953; 23(2): 121-31.
        [http://dx.doi.org/10.3109/17453675308991204] [PMID: 13138108]

[12]   Mazas FB. Guepar total knee prosthesis. Clin Orthop Relat Res 1973; (94): 211-21.
        [http://dx.doi.org/10.1097/00003086-197307000-00026] [PMID: 4743452]

[13]   Insall J, Scott WN, Ranawat CS. The total condylar knee prosthesis. A report of two hundred and twenty cases. J Bone Joint Surg Am 1979; 61(2): 173-80.
        [PMID: 422602]

[14]   Insall JN, Lachiewicz PF, Burstein AH. The posterior stabilized condylar prosthesis: a modification of the total condylar design. Two to four-year clinical experience. J Bone Joint Surg Am 1982; 64(9): 1317-23.
        [PMID: 7142239]

[15]   Scott RD. Duopatellar total knee replacement: the Brigham experience. Orthop Clin North Am 1982; 13(1): 89-102.
        [PMID: 7063201]

[16]   Insall JN, Clarke HD. Historic development, classification and characteristics of knee prostheses. In: Insall JN, Scott WN, Eds. Surgery of the Knee. 3rd ed. Churchill Livingstone 2001; Vol. 2.

[17]   Mont MA, Booth RE Jr, Laskin RS, *et al.* The spectrum of prosthesis design for primary total knee arthroplasty. Instr Course Lect 2003; 52: 397-407.
        [PMID: 12690866]

[18]   Maruyama S, Yoshiya S, Matsui N, Kuroda R, Kurosaka M. Functional comparison of posterior cruciate-retaining *versus* posterior stabilized total knee arthroplasty. J Arthroplasty 2004; 19(3): 349-53.
        [http://dx.doi.org/10.1016/j.arth.2003.09.010] [PMID: 15067650]

[19]   Clark CR, Rorabeck CH, MacDonald S, MacDonald D, Swafford J, Cleland D. Posterior-stabilized and cruciate-retaining total knee replacement: a randomized study. Clin Orthop Relat Res 2001; (392): 208-12.
[http://dx.doi.org/10.1097/00003086-200111000-00025] [PMID: 11716384]

[20]   Jacobs WC, Clement DJ, Wymenga AB. Retention *versus* removal of the posterior cruciate ligament in total knee replacement: a systematic literature review within the Cochrane framework. Acta Orthop 2005; 76(6): 757-68.
[http://dx.doi.org/10.1080/17453670510045345] [PMID: 16470427]

[21]   Shoji H, Wolf A, Packard S, Yoshino S. Cruciate retained and excised total knee arthroplasty. A comparative study in patients with bilateral total knee arthroplasty. Clin Orthop Relat Res 1994; (305): 218-22.
[PMID: 8050232]

[22]   Callaghan JJ, Insall JN, Greenwald AS, *et al.* Mobile-bearing knee replacement: concepts and results. Instr Course Lect 2001; (50): 431-449 35.

[23]   Huang CH, Liau JJ, Cheng CK. Fixed or mobile-bearing total knee arthroplasty. J Orthop Surg 2007; 2: 1.
[http://dx.doi.org/10.1186/1749-799X-2-1] [PMID: 17204165]

[24]   Buechel FF Sr, Buechel FF Jr, Pappas MJ. Eighteen-year evaluation of cementless meniscal bearing total ankle replacements. Instr Course Lect 2002; 51: 143-51.
[PMID: 12064099]

[25]   Buechel FF Sr, Buechel FF Jr, Pappas MJ, Dalessio J. Twenty-year evaluation of the New Jersey LCS Rotating Platform Knee Replacement. J Knee Surg 2002; 15(2): 84-9.
[PMID: 12013078]

[26]   Jordan LR, Olivo JL, Voorhorst PE. Survivorship analysis of cementless meniscal bearing total knee arthroplasty. Clin Orthop Relat Res 1997; (338): 119-23.
[http://dx.doi.org/10.1097/00003086-199705000-00018] [PMID: 9170372]

[27]   Scuderi GR. Revision total knee arthroplasty: how much constraint is enough? Clin Orthop Relat Res 2001; (392): 300-5.
[http://dx.doi.org/10.1097/00003086-200111000-00039] [PMID: 11716400]

[28]   Rosenberg AG, Verner JJ, Galante JO. Clinical results of total knee revision using the Total Condylar III prosthesis. Clin Orthop Relat Res 1991; (273): 83-90.
[PMID: 1959291]

[29]   Donaldson WF III, Sculco TP, Insall JN, Ranawat CS. Total condylar III knee prosthesis. Long-term follow-up study. Clin Orthop Relat Res 1988; (226): 21-8.
[PMID: 3335096]

[30]   Barrack RL. Evolution of the rotating hinge for complex total knee arthroplasty. Clin Orthop Relat Res 2001; (392): 292-9.
[http://dx.doi.org/10.1097/00003086-200111000-00038] [PMID: 11716398]

[31]   Kester MA, Cook SD, Harding AF, Rodriguez RP, Pipkin CS. An evaluation of the mechanical failure modalities of a rotating hinge knee prosthesis. Clin Orthop Relat Res 1988; (228): 156-63.

[PMID: 3342560]

[32] Barrack RL, Lyons TR, Ingraham RQ, Johnson JC. The use of a modular rotating hinge component in salvage revision total knee arthroplasty. J Arthroplasty 2000; 15(7): 858-66.
[http://dx.doi.org/10.1054/arth.2000.9056] [PMID: 11061445]

[33] Westrich GH, Mollano AV, Sculco TP, Buly RL, Laskin RS, Windsor R. Rotating hinge total knee arthroplasty in severely affected knees. Clin Orthop Relat Res 2000; (379): 195-208.
[http://dx.doi.org/10.1097/00003086-200010000-00023] [PMID: 11039807]

[34] Long WJ, Scuderi GR. High-flexion total knee arthroplasty. J Arthroplasty 2008; 23: 6-10 20.

[35] Luo SX, Su W, Zhao JM, Sha K, Wei QJ, Li XF. High-flexion vs conventional prostheses total knee arthroplasty: a meta-analysis. J Arthroplasty 2011; 26: 847-854 21.

[36] Sumino T, Gadikota HR, Varadarajan KM, Kwon YM, Rubash HE, Li G. Do high flexion posterior stabilised total knee arthroplasty designs increase knee flexion? A meta analysis. Int Orthop 2011; 35(9): 1309-19.
[http://dx.doi.org/10.1007/s00264-011-1228-4] [PMID: 21409370]

[37] Poilvache PL, Insall JN, Scuderi GR, Font-Rodriguez DE. Rotational landmarks and sizing of the distal femur in total knee arthroplasty. Clin Orthop Relat Res 1996; (331): 35-46.
[http://dx.doi.org/10.1097/00003086-199610000-00006] [PMID: 8895617]

[38] Chin KR, Dalury DF, Zurakowski D, Scott RD. Intraoperative measurements of male and female distal femurs during primary total knee arthroplasty. J Knee Surg 2002; 15(4): 213-7.
[PMID: 12416902]

[39] Hitt K, Shurman JR II, Greene K, *et al.* Anthropometric measurements of the human knee: correlation to the sizing of current knee arthroplasty systems. J Bone Joint Surg Am 2003; 85-A (Suppl. 4): 115-22.
[PMID: 14652402]

[40] Thomsen MG, Husted H, Bencke J, Curtis D, Holm G, Troelsen A. Do we need a gender-specific total knee replacement? A randomised controlled trial comparing a high-flex and a gender specific posterior design. J Bone Joint Surg Br 2012; 94: 787-792 23.

[41] Gender-specific knee replacements: a technology overview. J Am Acad Orthop Surg 2008; 16(2): 63-7.
[http://dx.doi.org/10.5435/00124635-200802000-00003] [PMID: 18252836]

[42] MacDonald SJ, Charron KD, Bourne RB, Naudie DD, McCalden RW, Rorabeck CH. The John Insall Award: gender-specific total knee replacement: prospectively collected clinical outcomes. Clin Orthop Relat Res 2008; 466(11): 2612-6.
[http://dx.doi.org/10.1007/s11999-008-0430-1] [PMID: 18800216]

[43] Canale ST, Beaty JH, Eds. Campbell's Operative Orthopaedics. 11th ed., St. Louis, Mo, USA: Mosby 2008.

[44] Hofmann AA, Plaster RL, Murdock LE. Subvastus (Southern) approach for primary total knee arthroplasty. Clin Orthop Relat Res 1991; (269): 70-7.
[PMID: 1864059]

[45]   Matsueda M, Gustilo RB. Subvastus and medial parapatellar approaches in total knee arthroplasty. Clin Orthop Relat Res 2000; (371): 161-8.
[http://dx.doi.org/10.1097/00003086-200002000-00020] [PMID: 10693563]

[46]   Engh GA, Holt BT, Parks NL. A midvastus muscle-splitting approach for total knee arthroplasty. J Arthroplasty 1997; 12(3): 322-31.
[http://dx.doi.org/10.1016/S0883-5403(97)90030-9] [PMID: 9113548]

[47]   Liu HW, Gu WD, Xu NW, Sun JY. Surgical approaches in total knee arthroplasty: a meta-analysis comparing the midvastus and subvastus to the medial parapatellar approach. J Arthroplasty 2014; 29(12): 2298-304.
[http://dx.doi.org/10.1016/j.arth.2013.10.023] [PMID: 24295800]

[48]   Keblish PA. The lateral approach to the valgus knee. Surgical technique and analysis of 53 cases with over two-year follow-up evaluation. Clin Orthop Relat Res 1991; (271): 52-62.
[PMID: 1914314]

[49]   Scuderi GR, Tenholder M, Capeci C. Surgical approaches in mini-incision total knee arthroplasty. Clin Orthop Relat Res 2004; (428): 61-7.
[http://dx.doi.org/10.1097/01.blo.0000148574.79874.d0] [PMID: 15534520]

[50]   Ritter MA, Faris PM, Keating EM, Meding JB. Postoperative alignment of total knee replacement. Its effect on survival. Clin Orthop Relat Res 1994; (299): 153-6.
[PMID: 8119010]

[51]   Krackow KA, Phillips MJ, Bayers-Thering M, Serpe L, Mihalko WM. Computer-assisted total knee arthroplasty: navigation in TKA. Orthopedics 2003; 26(10): 1017-23.
[PMID: 14577524]

[52]   Hetaimish BM, Khan MM, Simunovic N, Al-Harbi HH, Bhandari M, Zalzal PK. Meta-analysis of navigation *vs* conventional total knee arthroplasty. J Arthroplasty 2012; 27(6): 1177-82.
[http://dx.doi.org/10.1016/j.arth.2011.12.028] [PMID: 22333865]

[53]   Siston RA, Giori NJ, Goodman SB, Delp SL. Surgical navigation for total knee arthroplasty: a perspective. J Biomech 2007; 40: 728-735 83.

[54]   Burnett RS, Barrack RL. Computer-assisted total knee arthroplasty is currently of no proven clinical benefit: a systematic review. Clin Orthop Relat Res 2013; 471(1): 264-76.
[http://dx.doi.org/10.1007/s11999-012-2528-8] [PMID: 22948522]

[55]   Bae DK, Song SJ. Computer assisted navigation in knee arthroplasty. Clin Orthop Surg 2011; 3: 259-267 84.
[http://dx.doi.org/10.4055/cios.2011.3.4.259]

[56]   Victor J, Premanathan A. Virtual 3D planning and patient specific surgical guides for osteotomies around the knee: a feasibility and proof-of-concept study. Bone Joint J 2013; 95-B(11) (Suppl. A): 153-8.
[http://dx.doi.org/10.1302/0301-620X.95B11.32950] [PMID: 24187376]

[57]   Thienpont E, Schwab PE, Fennema P. A systematic review and meta-analysis of patient-specific instrumentation for improving alignment of the components in total knee replacement. Bone Joint J 2014; 96-B(8): 1052-61.

[http://dx.doi.org/10.1302/0301-620X.96B8.33747] [PMID: 25086121]

[58] Victor J, Dujardin J, Vandenneucker H, Arnout N, Bellemans J. Patient-specific guides do not improve accuracy in total knee arthroplasty: a prospective randomized controlled trial. Clin Orthop Relat Res 2014; 472(1): 263-71.
[http://dx.doi.org/10.1007/s11999-013-2997-4] [PMID: 23616267]

[59] Lustig S, Scholes CJ, Oussedik S, Coolican MR, Parker DA. Unsatisfactory accuracy with VISIONAIRE patient-specific cutting jigs for total knee arthroplasty. J Arthroplasty 2014; 29(1): 249-50.
[http://dx.doi.org/10.1016/j.arth.2013.05.020] [PMID: 23891059]

[60] Woolson ST, Harris AH, Wagner DW, Giori NJ. Component alignment during total knee arthroplasty with use of standard or custom instrumentation: a randomized clinical trial using computed tomography for postoperative alignment measurement. J Bone Joint Surg Am 2014; 96(5): 366-72.
[http://dx.doi.org/10.2106/JBJS.L.01722] [PMID: 24599197]

[61] Pakos EE, Ntzani EE, Trikalinos TA. Patellar resurfacing in total knee arthroplasty. A meta-analysis. J Bone Joint Surg Am 2005; 87(7): 1438-45.
[http://dx.doi.org/10.2106/JBJS.D.02422] [PMID: 15995109]

[62] Burnett RS, Haydon CM, Rorabeck CH, Bourne RB. Patella resurfacing *versus* nonresurfacing in total knee arthroplasty: results of a randomized controlled clinical trial at a minimum of 10 years followup. Clin Orthop Relat Res 2004; (428): 12-25.
[http://dx.doi.org/10.1097/01.blo.0000148594.05443.a3] [PMID: 15534514]

[63] Bourne RB, Burnett RS. The consequences of not resurfacing the patella. Clin Orthop Relat Res 2004; (428): 166-9.
[http://dx.doi.org/10.1097/01.blo.0000147137.05927.bf] [PMID: 15534538]

[64] Ranawat CS, Meftah M, Windsor EN, Ranawat AS. Cementless fixation in total knee arthroplasty: down the boulevard of broken dreams - affirms. J Bone Joint Surg Br 2012; 94(11) (Suppl. A): 82-4.
[http://dx.doi.org/10.1302/0301-620X.94B11.30826] [PMID: 23118389]

[65] Nakama GY, Peccin MS, Almeida GJ, Lira Neto OdeA, Queiroz AA, Navarro RD. Cemented, cementless or hybrid fixation options in total knee arthroplasty for osteoarthritis and other non-traumatic diseases. Cochrane Database Syst Rev 2012; 10: CD006193.
[http://dx.doi.org/10.1002/14651858.CD006193] [PMID: 23076921]

[66] Berger RA, Lyon JH, Jacobs JJ, *et al.* Problems with cementless total knee arthroplasty at 11 years followup. Clin Orthop Relat Res 2001; 196-207 68.
[http://dx.doi.org/10.1097/00003086-200111000-00024]

[67] Ezzet KA, Garcia R, Barrack RL. Effect of component fixation method on osteolysis in total knee arthroplasty. Clin Orthop Relat Res 1995; 86–91 69. Goldberg VM, Kraay M. The outcome of the cementless tibial component: a minimum 14-year clinical evaluation. Clin Orthop Relat Res 2004; 214-20.

[68] Cuckler JM. The infected total knee: management options. J Arthroplasty 2005; 20(4) (Suppl. 2): 33-6.
[http://dx.doi.org/10.1016/j.arth.2005.03.004] [PMID: 15991126]

[69] Hanssen AD, Rand JA, Osmon DR. Treatment of the infected total knee arthroplasty with insertion of

another prosthesis. The effect of antibiotic-impregnated bone cement. Clin Orthop Relat Res 1994; (309): 44-55.
[PMID: 7994976]

[70]   Rubash HE, Ed. Orthopaedic knowledge update: Hip and knee reconstruction 3. Rosemont, IL: American Academy of Orthopaedic Surgeons 2006; pp. 1-177.

[71]   McPherson EJ. Adult reconstruction, In Miller MD (ed): Re-view of Orthopaedics, ed 4th. Philadelphia, PA, Saunders (Elsevier), 2004, pp. 266-308.

[72]   Peters CL, Crofoot CD, Froimson MI. Knee reconstruction and replacement. In: Fischgrund JS, Ed. Orthopaedic Knowledge Update 9. Rosemont, IL: American Academy of Orthopaedic Surgeons 2008; pp. 457-71.

[73]   Ranawat CS, Flynn WF Jr, Saddler S, Hansraj KK, Maynard MJ. Long-term results of the total condylar knee arthroplasty. A 15-year survivorship study. Clin Orthop Relat Res 1993; (286): 94-102.
[PMID: 8425373]

[74]   Borus T, Thornhill T. Unicompartmental knee arthroplasty. J Am Acad Orthop Surg 2008; 16(1): 9-18.
[http://dx.doi.org/10.5435/00124635-200801000-00003] [PMID: 18180388]

[75]   Laurencin CT, Zelicof SB, Scott RD, Ewald FC. Unicompartmental versus total knee arthroplasty in the same patient. A comparative study. Clin Orthop Relat Res 1991; (273): 151-6.
[PMID: 1959264]

[76]   The Australian National Joint Replacement Registry. Annual Report 2012. Available at: https://aoanjrr.dmac.adelaide.edu.au/annual-reports-2012. Accessed August 12, 2013.

[77]   The National Joint Registry of England, Wales and Northern Ireland. 9th Annual Report 2012. Available at: http://www.njrcentre.org.uk/njrcentre/Portals/0/Documents/England/Reports/9th_annual_report/NJR%209th%20Annual%20Report%202012.pdf. Accessed September 22, 2013.

[78]   Inacio MC, Paxton EW, Dillon MT. Understanding Orthopaedic Registry Studies: A Comparison with Clinical Studies. J Bone Joint Surg Am 2016; 98(1): e3.
[http://dx.doi.org/10.2106/JBJS.N.01332] [PMID: 26738910]

CHAPTER 9

Role of Cartilage Surgery and Hip Arthroscopy in the Management of Early Hip Arthritis: Current Concepts

R. Papalia[1]**, R. Zini**[2]**, B. Zampogna**[1]**, V. Denaro**[1] **and N. Maffulli**[3,4,*]

[1] *Department of Orthopaedic and Trauma Surgery, Campus Biomedico University of Rome, Via Alvaro del Portillo 200, Rome, Italy*

[2] *Department of Orthopaedic and Trauma Surgery, Villa Maria Cecilia Hospital, GVM Care & Research, Via Corriera 1, 48010 Cotignola, Ravenna, Italy*

[3] *Department of Musculoskeletal Disorders, Faculty of Medicine and Surgery, University of Salerno, 84081 Baronissi, Salerno, Italy*

[4] *Centre for Sports and Exercise Medicine, Barts and The London School of Medicine and Dentistry, Mile End Hospital, 275 Bancroft Road, London E1 4DG, England*

Abstract: The main aim of cartilage surgery and hip arthroscopy in the management of early hip arthritis is to avoid conversion to total hip arthroplasty, and the earlier the treatment, the greater is the possibility to achieve this purpose. Several techniques have been proposed, such as microfracture, simple debridement, and autologous chondrocyte implantation-matrix assisted autologous chondrocyte implantation (ACI-MACI) for arthroscopic approach and open ACI-MACI and mosaicplasty for open surgery. Arthroscopic debridement associated with microfracture, depending on the patient's condition, represents the best choice for the treatment of early stages osteoarthritis (OA) of the hip joint, especially where an associated chondral defect has to be fixed. The cause of OA must be promptly individuated and the cartilage surgery must always be associated (except for degenerative OA) with procedures aimed to fix any other structural defect in order to avoid further degeneration and to improve the outcome of the surgery.

* **Corresponding author Nicola Maffulli:** Centre for Sports and Exercise Medicine, Barts and The London School of Medicine and Dentistry, Mile End Hospital, 275 Bancroft Road, London E1 4DG, England; Tel: + 44 20 8223 8839; Fax: + 44 20 8223 8930; E-mail: n.maffulli@qmul.ac.uk

Keywords: Articular cartilage repair, Autologous chondrocyte implantation, Cartilage surgery, Debridement, Hip arthroscopy, Hip chondral lesion, Hip osteoarthritis, Microfracture, Mosaicplasty, Open hip surgery, Osteochondral allograft transplantation.

CHONDRAL DISEASE OF THE HIP JOINT, LESIONS AND CLASSIFICATIONS

The pelvis, and the hip region in particular, are some of the most relevant weight-bearing surfaces of the body, and this is one of the reasons for progressive overload of the hip cartilage in adults as well as in younger subjects involved in athletics, jumping sports, or other high demanding physical activities [1]. The overload of the joint is a common feature of the disease for both elderly and young people, but while the former are more likely to be affected by a degenerative disease, the latter usually have an underlying mechanical cause that provides pathological shearing of the cartilage or altered articular structures that leads to instability, femoral-acetabular impingement (either cam or pincer impingement), and focal cartilage overload. The main causes of hip pathology in the young adult are developmental dysplasia, Perthes disease [1], collagen deficiency syndromes (Marfan's disease, ochronosis) and coxa valga, while trauma, labral tears, autoimmune disorders, osteonecrosis and Paget's disease are more commonly diagnosed in the elderly [1]. A specific kind of chondral injury which may lead to further development of arthritis is the so called "lateral impact injury" [2] (lateral trauma on the greater trochanter), which results in chondral defects of the labrum and/or of the femoral head. The site of the first cartilage insult is termed as "Watershed zone" [3] and if this site is near the labrochondral junction, it is more likely that the surrounding cartilage develops arthritis because of destabilization. The cause of osteoarthritis (OA) or of the cartilage defect must be assessed clearly and addressed before selecting the patient for surgery, in order to treat the defect in its totality and not aiming to relieve the symptoms only. Tönnis classification is utilized to assess the OA degree in plain radiographs, while surgically, the Outerbridge classification is commonly used to define the grade of hip chondral disease in direct arthroscopic view. Grade I has been described as softening and swelling of the cartilage, Grades II and III involve proper lesions and fragmentation of the tissue, and Grade IV refers to subchondral bone exposure. The following tables (Tables **1** and **2**) summarize these classifications for the hip joint.

Table 1. The Tönnis classification.

Grade	Description
0	No osteoarthritis.
1	Increased sclerosis, slight narrowing of the joint space, no or slight loss of head sphericity.
2	Small cysts, moderate narrowing of the joint space, moderate loss of head sphericity.
3	Large cysts, severe narrowing or obliteration of the joint space, severe deformity of the head.

Table 2. The Outerbridge classification.

Grade	Size	Description
I		Softening/swelling
II	≤1.3 cm (1/2 inch)	Fragmentation/fissuring
III	>1.3 cm (1/2 inch)	
IV		Erosion/subchondral bone exposure

Talking about early OA, one should take into consideration Grades 1-2 of the Tönnis classification or I-II of the Outerbridge classification. The main aim in arthroscopic or open treatment of early hip chondral defects is to avoid the conversion to total hip arthroplasty (THA), and the earlier the surgery, the greater is the possibility of success in this regard. Before arthroscopic evaluation, the first view in imaging (mainly radiography and MRI) using Tönnis classification may be a potential predictor of success of the surgery, since it has been reported that the narrowing extent (<2mm) strongly predicts the conversion to THA. Moreover, the early detection of cam or pincer impingement can lead to a prompt treatment of these defects, through debridement of the spurs, in order to stop further progression of OA.

MORPHOLOGICAL FINDINGS IN EARLY ARTHRITIS

Early arthritis usually affects the surface cartilage of the femoral head and the acetabular labrum; sometimes the acetabular fossa can also be involved. Technically speaking, a labral tear is not a proper form of arthritis, although it leads to chronic instability, which constitutes the cause of arthritis itself. This is the reason why the labral tear is the most frequently associated lesion. It is suspected clinically by groin pain and clicking sound during the movement of the hip. It can be easily individualized arthroscopically while viewing the central compartment and localized in the superior quadrant. The labrum has a central vascular zone (attached to the acetabulum) and an avascular free edge, and the arrangement is similar to meniscus in the knee [2]. Consequently, the tears can be found more likely in the edge. Chondral lesions of the surface cartilage of the femoral head can be also seen with a direct view of the central compartment. The size and the kind of lesions can be assessed through the Outerbridge classification, and in the early disease, they should not exceed 1.3 cm in width. Another type of damage is delamination of the cartilage from the underlying subchondral bone, often with the risk of this cartilage becoming a loose body if it breaks.

INDICATIONS AND TECHNIQUES IN ARTHROSCOPIC SURGERY

Labral Tears (Figs. 1, 2): As already mentioned, labral edge tears are the most frequent lesions found, and the treatment can be resection (in order to provide the labrum with a new plain rim) or repair. It has been demonstrated that the repair of the labrum leads to later onset of hip arthritis [2, 4]. Therefore, the labrum should always be repaired in either Tönnis Grade 0 or in 1-2, which serves both a curative and a preventive role. The labral edge tear is often accompanied by the detachment of labrum from the acetabulum, which can be treated by insertion of the suture anchors. However the procedure is technically demanding because of the need for correct placement of the anchor with a diverging orientation in order to avoid the acetabular articular surface.

Chondral Lesions (Fig. 3): Debridement is the most common treatment for chondral defects, especially in low-grade arthritis. Since the grade of the lesion significantly affects the outcome of surgery [2], it is necessary to act as early as possible, when the patient can be a candidate for the surgery.

• Simple **Debridement (Fig. 4)** of the joint surfaces is carried out through the use of a shaver, in order to regularize the damaged cartilage and provide a smooth shearing surface for the movement of the joint. Results have demonstrated that

30 to 60% of patients undergoing debridement reported good postoperative clinical outcomes and significantly delayed the conversion to THA [5].

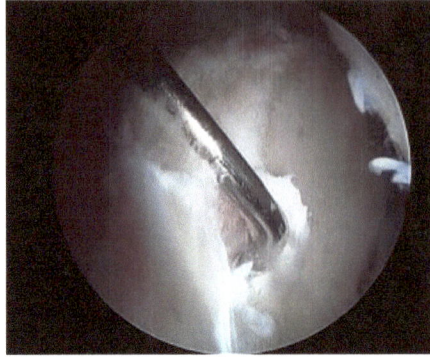

Fig. (1). Labrum tears evaluation.

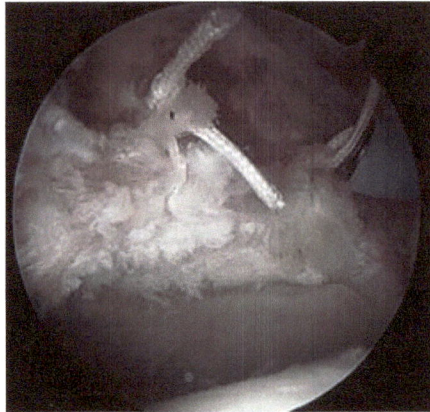

Fig. (2). Labrum repair.

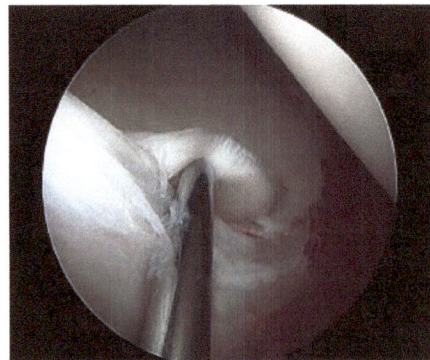

Fig. (3). Acetabular chondral lesion.

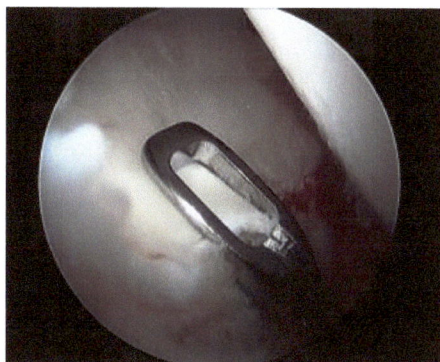

Fig. (4). Debridement of the joint surfaces and flap removal.

One of the most affirmed and common treatments is the microfracture technique, which is indicated in low-grade OA with associated focal lesions of maximum 4 cm^2 area [6].

- **Microfracture:** Involves digging some holes with an awl, perpendicular to the cartilage surface, with a diameter of about 4 mm, leaving the same space between each hole (4 mm). In this way, bleeding of the trabecular bone occurs and marrow cells together with growth factors reach the injured surface in order to heal the defect. It is reported in the literature that microfracture provides healing of small lesions (between 1.5 and 3 cm^2) in more than 90% cases [7, 8] with a microscopically good-quality cartilage. Conversely, it has been demonstrated to be of little effectiveness in Tönnis Grade 3 or Outerbridge 3-4 lesions [6].

Another effective treatment these days is ACI [6]. This technique can be carried out only if certain conditions are satisfied that include the following: the lesion must be a full thickness tear and the subchondral bone must be intact. Lesions larger than 3 cm but smaller than 10 cm can be treated in this fashion.

- **The ACI-MACI (Figs. 5-8):** Technique is performed with the help of a biology laboratory, because of the need for a culture-based growth of the chondrocytes harvested from a joint (other than the involved hip) of the patient. Once the cultivated chondrocytes have grown enough to fill the lesion, they are implanted. Latest updates in this technique involve the use of a scaffold (d hip) o) (hence

MACI, "matrix-assisted ACI") to set the correct delivery of the cells on the lesion [6]. This technique can be performed arthroscopically, in contrast with simple ACI (in which a patch and an injectable solution are used). Although this technique may be considered a shared option for the treatment of mild to severe lesions, it has not been demonstrated significantly better than simple debridement for either early or later grades of OA.

Management of the cartilage delamination can involve both these techniques, once the less damaged portion of the defect is removed. However, it has been reported that direct suture or fibrin adhesion could also be provided for small lesions if the delaminated cartilage appears healthy [9 - 11].

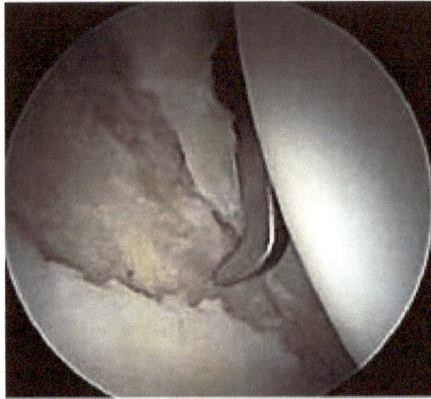

Fig. (5). Acetabular chondral lesion.

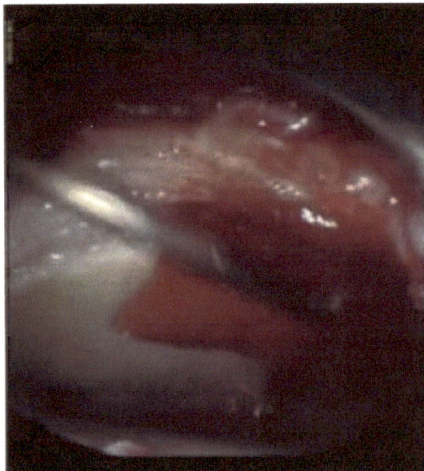

Fig. (6). ACI implant for acetabular chondral lesion.

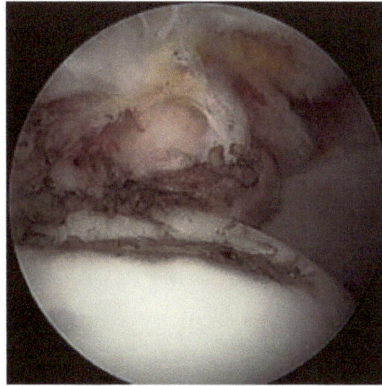

Fig. (7). Femoral head chondral lesion.

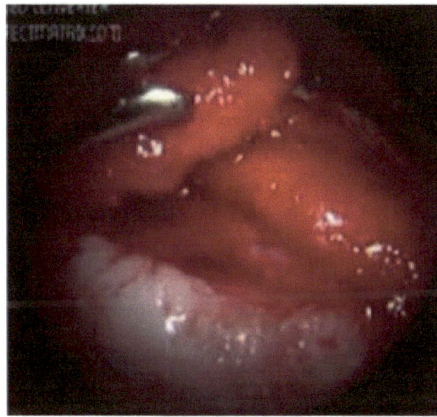

Fig. (8). ACI implant for femoral head chondral lesion.

INDICATIONS AND TECHNIQUES IN OPEN CARTILAGE SURGERY

Open surgery is gradually fading out and making way for the most affirmed, simple, and less invasive arthroscopy. Nevertheless, in selected cases, open surgery can still be used if there is a technical impediment or in cases where the micro invasive technique is truly demanding.

• **The ACI-MACI:** Treatment described in the previous paragraph is one of the cases in which open surgery still finds some application. As already explained, only MACI can be performed arthroscopically, while the standard ACI technique is performed through direct access to the hip joint, dislocation of the femoral head, and implantation of a patch to contain the injectable chondrocyte-based solution. Complication of this technique involves infection at the donor site and osteonecrosis of the femoral head, due to the dislocation. In fact, the technique is approved in Europe, but not in the United States [6].

Another open therapeutic option for femoral head defects is mosaicplasty, which is indicated in young adults with no or early OA and lesions with maximum thickness smaller than 3 cm^2.

- **Mosaicplasty:** Involves transplantation of cylindrical bone and cartilage autografts, harvested from another healthy joint and directly implanted in the damaged joint surface. Sometimes they can also be harvested from the inferolateral aspect of the involved femur. This kind of surgery requires surgical dislocation of the hip joint. Excellent results have been reported with a 30-month follow-up, reporting a THA conversion of 0% [12].

Osteochondral allograft transplantation is quite similar to mosaicplasty and is indicated in small lesions as well. The osteochondral cylinders are conversely harvested from a cadaver. Very few studies have reported good outcomes for this procedure for the hip joint.

FINAL CONSIDERATION ABOUT THE TREATMENT OF EARLY HIP ARTHRITIS

Several types of techniques have been highlighted in the study, in order to provide a thorough overview of hip surgery. The challenge for the surgeon is to select the correct patient for the best treatment. The following consideration of the authors may be helpful in discerning the proper utility of different surgeries. First, microfracture should be considered as the best arthroscopic treatment for small size lesions, with a success rate that may rise up to 90%. This is the reason for the worldwide spread and frequent use of this procedure. However, some comparisons reported in the literature showed that patients treated by MACI technique achieved significantly better results than others treated with simple debridement.

Concerning cartilage surgery, comparable results were reported for any kind of cartilage transplantation procedure, but it must be taken into account that if the MACI technique requires sophisticated support facilities for culturing chondrocytes and the need for at least two surgeries for harvesting and implantation, mosaicplasty is simpler and sometimes can be performed on one joint only, using a healthy site of cartilage of the same joint for harvesting. Moreover, the conditions of the subchondral bone must also be considered when a chondrocyte transplantation surgery is to be approached. As explained previously, in order to perform a chondral transplant, there is a need for a healthy subchondral bone, a condition that cannot be ignored. In these cases, mosaicplasty or allogeneic osteochondral transplant have a strong indication. One of the factors worth mentioning is the cost-effectiveness of the procedure.

Debridement and the microfracture technique are considered easier and cheaper ones, because they do not need special instrumentation (both can be properly performed with a standard arthroscopic surgical set) and no supportive or associated procedures are required. Mosaicplasty is also a cost-effective technique, especially if a single joint is involved. Even then, because of the major technical difficulty of the procedure, it could require longer operative time and special tools for the harvesting of the cylinders.

MACI is obviously the more complex and expensive technique, because of the laboratory support procedures involved in this kind of surgery and the need for two different procedures. To sum up, the authors wish to advise that arthroscopic debridement associated with microfracture is the best choice for the treatment of early-stage OA of the hip joint, especially where an associated chondral defect has to be fixed. The other techniques are usually performed at specialized centers and reserved for selected patients with severe associated conditions, such as chondromalacia, osteomalacia, or other pathologies involving bone and cartilage.

Arthroscopic treatment provides better results and must be preferred to open surgery, depending on the patient's conditions. It is worth reiterating that the cause of OA must be promptly individualized and cartilage surgery must always be associated (except for degenerative OA) with procedures aimed to fix any other structural defect, in order to avoid further degeneration and to improve the outcome of the surgery in future.

CONFLICT OF INTEREST

The authors confirm that the authors have no conflict of interest to declare for this publication.

ACKNOWLEDGEMENTS

Declared none.

REFERENCES

[1]   Parvizi J, Leunig M, Ganz R. Femoroacetabular impingement. J Am Acad Orthop Surg 2007; 15(9): 561-70.
       [http://dx.doi.org/10.5435/00124635-200709000-00006] [PMID: 17761612]

[2]   Khanduja V, Villar RN. Arthroscopic surgery of the hip: current concepts and recent advances. J Bone Joint Surg Br 2006; 88(12): 1557-66.
       [http://dx.doi.org/10.1302/0301-620X.88B12.18584] [PMID: 17159164]

[3]   McCarthy JC, Noble PC, Schuck MR, Wright J, Lee J. The watershed labral lesion: its relationship to early arthritis of the hip. J Arthroplasty 2001; 16(8) (Suppl. 1): 81-7.
       [http://dx.doi.org/10.1054/arth.2001.28370] [PMID: 11742456]

[4]   Espinosa N, Rothenfluh DA, Beck M, Ganz R, Leunig M. Treatment of femoro-acetabular impingement: preliminary results of labral refixation. J Bone Joint Surg Am 2006; 88(5): 925-35.
       [http://dx.doi.org/10.2106/JBJS.E.00290] [PMID: 16651565]

[5]   Farjo LA, Glick JM, Sampson TG. Hip arthroscopy for acetabular labral tears. Arthroscopy 1999; 15(2): 132-7.
       [PMID: 10210068] [http://dx.doi.org/10.1053/ar.1999.v15.015013]

[6]   El Bitar YF, Lindner D, Jackson TJ, Domb BG. Joint-preserving surgical options for management of chondral injuries of the hip. J Am Acad Orthop Surg 2014; 22(1): 46-56.
       [http://dx.doi.org/10.5435/JAAOS-22-01-46] [PMID: 24382879]

[7]   Karthikeyan S, Roberts S, Griffin D. Microfracture for acetabular chondral defects in patients with femoroacetabular impingement: results at second-look arthroscopic surgery. Am J Sports Med 2012; 40(12): 2725-30.
       [http://dx.doi.org/10.1177/0363546512465400] [PMID: 23136178]

[8]   Philippon MJ, Schenker ML, Briggs KK, Maxwell RB. Can microfracture produce repair tissue in acetabular chondral defects? Arthroscopy 2008; 24(1): 46-50.
       [http://dx.doi.org/10.1016/j.arthro.2007.07.027] [PMID: 18182201]

[9]   Sekiya JK, Martin RL, Lesniak BP. Arthroscopic repair of delaminated acetabular articular cartilage in femoroacetabular impingement. Orthopedics 2009; 32(9): orthosupersite.com/view.asp?rID=42859.
       [http://dx.doi.org/10.3928/01477447-20090728-44] [PMID: 19750994]

[10]   Stafford GH, Bunn JR, Villar RN. Arthroscopic repair of delaminated acetabular articular cartilage using fibrin adhesive. Results at one to three years. Hip Int J Clin 2011; 21(6): 744-50.

[PMID: 22117261]

[11]   Tzaveas AP, Villar RN. Arthroscopic repair of acetabular chondral delamination with fibrin adhesive. Hip Int 2010; 20(1): 115-9.
[PMID: 20235074]

[12]   Girard J, Roumazeille T, Sakr M, Migaud H. Osteochondral mosaicplasty of the femoral head. Hip Int 2011; 21(5): 542-8.
[http://dx.doi.org/10.5301/HIP.2011.8659] [PMID: 21948031]

CHAPTER 10

Total Hip Arthroplasty-evolution and Current Concepts

J.V. Srinivas [*] and **Mohan Puttaswamy**

Fortis Hospital, Bannerghatta Road, Bangalore, India

Abstract: Total hip arthroplasty (THA) has been designated as the Operation of the century. The past 3-4 decades have seen tremendous improvement in the patient outcomes, products and technology that has enabled all these changes to improve the quality of life of our patients with problems of the hip joint. We have reviewed the surgical approaches to the hip joint, the bearing surfaces, implant selection and their problems and complications in this chapter. We have also stated our approach and philosophy to have good outcome of THA.

Keywords: Approaches to the hip, Bearing surfaces, Cemented arthroplasty, Deep vein thrombosis, Dislocation of the hip, Total Hip Arthroplasty, Uncemented arthroplasty, Wear.

INTRODUCTION

Total hip arthroplasty has a rich history of innovation and some have rightly called it the "Operation of the century". The earliest total hip replacement goes back to 1891 where Professor Themistocles Gluck presented the use of ivory to replace femoral head for post tubercular arthritis. Along the way there were attempts by Smith-Peterson with his "mold arthroplasty" using glass in 1925 and then went onto Stainless steel as a material of choice in his later generation prosthesis. Meanwhile, the true revolution in joint replacement is attributed to Sir John Charnley, who worked at the Manchester Royal Infirmary and developed the

[*] **Corresponding author JV Srinivas:** 154/9, Bannerghatta Road, Opposite IIM-B, Bengaluru, Karnataka-560076, Bangalore, India; Tel/Fax: 080-66214121; E-mails: mohanortho@gmail.com, jvsrinivas72@gmail.com

Ashish Anand (Ed.)

principle of "Low Friction Arthroplasty" in the early 1960's and thus heralded the revolution in joint replacement surgery.

Surgical Approaches to Total Hip Arthroplasty (THA)

There are many surgical approaches which have been described for performing THA. The approach is primarily determined by surgical training, perceived advantage and disadvantage of each approach and surgeon familiarity with each approach. Broadly, surgical approaches in THA can be divided as posterior, lateral and anterior approaches. In posterior approach the abductor mechanism of the hip is not violated and posterior capsule is divided and arthroplasty performed. The primary criticism of this approach is the higher incidence of dislocation in comparison to other approaches. Lateral or antero-lateral approach in some way or other violates the abductor mechanism and thus has the disadvantage of potentially disturbing the main motor of the hip joint and could lead to long term issues if there is no healing of the abductor mechanism. Direct anterior approach is a true inter-nervous approach with minimal disruption to the hip musculature and thus leading to a better early recovery than other approaches. Having said that a well performed THA by any approach will generally result in a good clinical outcome; the idea should be to tailor the approach to a given clinical situation.

Posterior Approach

This is the most commonly used approach for performing THA. The advantages of this approach is, it is the most commonly used and taught approach. The basic premise of this approach is that the Gluteus Maximus is split and the hip joint approached just posterior to the Gluteus medius tendon (Fig. **1**). The other advantage is that there is no disruption of in the abductor mechanism of the hip joint while the disadvantage is a higher dislocation rate in comparison to the lateral, anterolateral or the anterior approach.

The lateral approach to total hip arthroplasty has numerous modifications which go by eponymous names as described by its authors. But, it suffices to mention that all these approaches in some form or another involve damage to the abductor mechanism of the hip joint. The most widely used approach is the Hardinge approach, where the Gluteus medius and the Vastus lateralis are taken in a single lazy J incision and an anterior dislocation of the hip performed. This approach can be performed either with the patient supine or in the lateral position. The disadvantage of this approach is that if dissection extends 5 cm proximal to the tip of the trochanter it could end up damaging the Superior gluteal nerve and leading to a limp clinically.

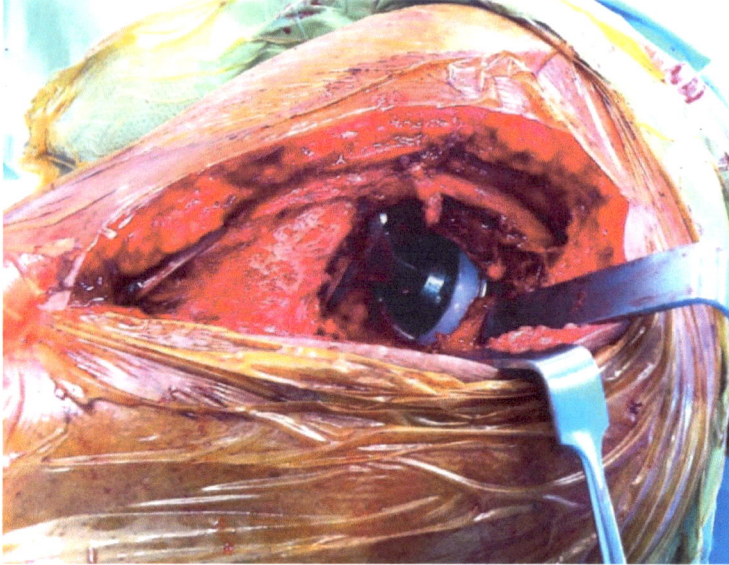

Fig. (1). The approach is just posterior to the gluteus medius tendon.

Direct anterior approach to THA *has off late taken* the fancy of arthroplasty surgeons. This approach has been described long time ago, where the patient is positioned supine and approached by an inter-nervous plane involving the femoral and Superior gluteal nerve. The plane is developed between the TFL and the Sartorius superficially and Gluteus medius and Rectus femoris in the deeper plane (Fig. **2**). The advantage of this approach is early mobilization, earlier restoration of gait kinematics and lesser dislocation rates. The disadvantages of this approach is *the* difficulty *to* access femoral canal, which *needs* special equipment like offset broaches, reamers and some surgeons use a specialized table for this approach.

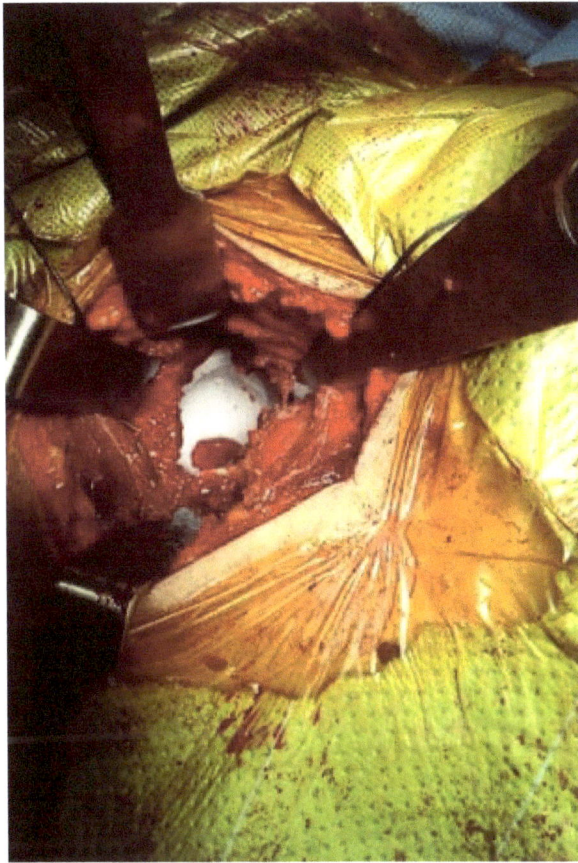

Fig. (2). Direct anterior approach showing the method of positioning the retractors.

Surgical Approaches During Revision Total Hip Replacement

Revision total hip replacement poses certain unique challenges where the existing components have to be removed with minimal loss of bone and also give adequate access to perform extensive reconstruction. Most surgeons use a variation of the posterior approach to perform their revision surgery. It can be combined with trochanteric slide, conventional trochanteric osteotomy or an extended trochanteric osteotomy with little additional damage to the abductor mechanism. Trochanteric Slide is a procedure where the Gluteus Medius, Vastus Lateralis are taken together as a sleeve along with a 1cm thick bone fragment from the greater trochanter and after the surgery reattached to the existing bony bed with bone to bone healing. Conventional trochanteric Osteotomy consists of reflecting the entire abductor mechanism of the hip proximally and the most important advantage is that it does not damage the Superior gluteal nerve. The problems with this approach is that adequate thickness of bone has to be taken for bone to bone healing and if the flap is too thick it might compromise the lateral support for the femoral stem. There is a higher chance of non-union and "trochanteric escape" proximally. It needs to be reattached with Cables or Trochanteric claw plate. Schutzer SF *et al.* reported a 97% union rate with a 3 or 4 wire reattachment technique [1]. To avoid the problems of reattachment and non-union of the conventional trochanteric osteotomy Extended Greater Trochanteric Osteotomy (ETO) was developed and has proven to be a very important modification in revision total hip arthroplasty (Figs. **3**, **4**). It has some useful advantages like *giving* access to the entire femoral canal to remove implant or cement, has a high union rate as there is a large bony contact area. Most series show greater than 95% union rate in ETO technique. Huffman *et al.* reported 100% union rate for ETO in 43 hips after using this technique [2].

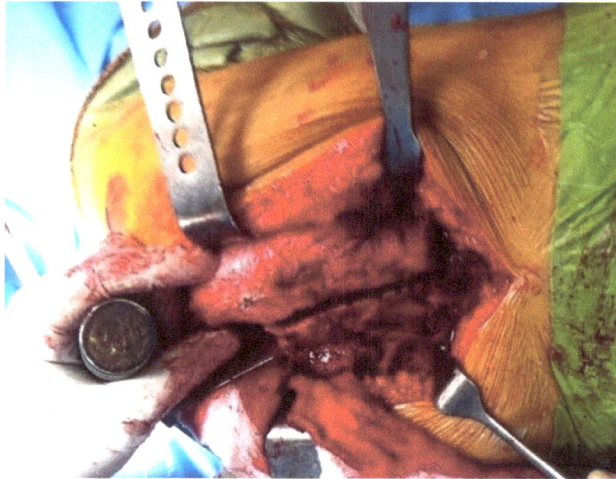

Fig. (3). Intraoperative image of posterior approach ETO.

Bearing Surfaces in THA

There has been broadly 2 schools of thoughts in the development of bearing surfaces "Hard on Hard" bearings and "Hard on Soft" bearing surfaces. In the 1960's Mackee and Ring introduced the metal on metal implants and in 1970's Boutin developed ceramic on ceramic bearing surfaces which represents the hard on hard school of thought; Dr. John Charnley developed the hard on soft bearing with his metal on polyethylene bearing in the 1960's and with his concept of "low friction arthroplasty"- a new era of total hip arthroplasty was born.

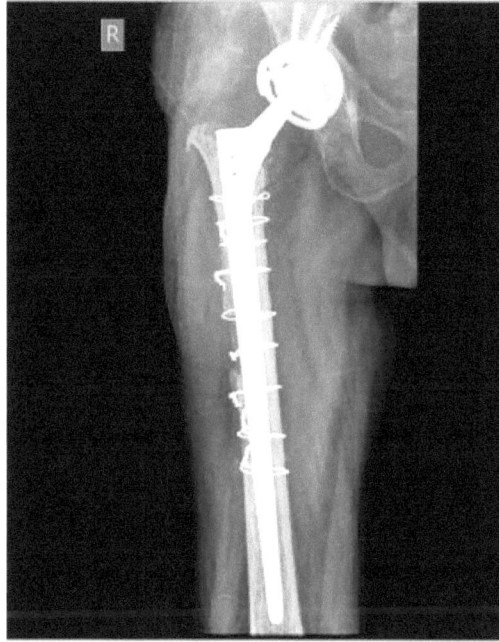

Fig. (4). X ray image of a healed HTO after fixation with cables.

Tribology is defined as the science and technology of interacting surfaces in relative motion. The "Low friction" principle helps to reduce the shear forces across the joint surface and thus prevents early loosening and aids in implant survivorship.

Hard on Soft Bearings

The classic- most widely used bearing surface in the world is the Metal (Cobalt Chrome) on Ultra High Molecular Weight Polyethylene (UHMWPE). The advantages of this bearing surface are its cost effectiveness, absence of squeaking and bearing related Metal ion complications. The experience of the last 5 decades has made this the most attractive of bearing options. UHMWPE was first used in the 1960's and the early problems were wear related. The problem of polyethylene wear was initially referred to as "cement disease" [3] thinking that it was related to the cement particles. Later it was found to be due to the particle induced chronic inflammatory response leading to bone resorption and osteolysis. This ultimately led to peri-prosthetic osteolysis and aseptic loosening. This phenomenon is noticed when the wear rates are more than 0.1mm/year. When the wear rates are less than 0.05mm/year minimal osteolysis is seen [4]. Highly cross linked polyethylene (XLPE) was introduced clinically in the year 1998 and had a dramatic reduction in the wear rates. Beksac and Dorr have shown that the usage of highly cross linked polyethylene as liner has shown significant reduction in wear rates compared to conventional polyethylene [5, 6]. Meanwhile, the early polyethylene liners had the problem of oxidation due to gamma sterilization in air which had further degradation when stored for a long period of time. To address the issue of oxidation and free radical generation a few strategies were devised like annealing, re-melting and infusion with Vitamin E. Re-melting the polyethylene is associated with decrease of mechanical property of the liner while annealing will still leave a few free radicals in the polyethylene [7]. Table **1** shows that there is a decrease of the wear rates in XLPE in comparison to conventional PE and in a meta-analysis by Kurtz *et al.* [8] they showed that the pooled odds ratio for the risk of osteolysis in HXLPE *versus* conventional liners was 0.13 (95% confidence interval, 0.06–0.27) among studies with minimum 5-year follow up which *equals* 87% reduction in the chances of having osteolysis.

Table 1. Polyethylene penetration in highly cross linked *versus* conventional polyethylene.

Study	2D Linear Penetration Conventional Poly*	2D Linear Penetration XLPE*
Beksac 2009 (5)	0.002	0.12
Dorr 2005(6)	0.065	0.029
Kurtz 2011(8)	0.042	0.137

*All measurements are in mm/year

Hard on Hard Bearing Surfaces

Ceramic on Ceramic Bearing (C on C)

The alumina on alumina ceramic bearing exhibit certain unique properties like low wear rates due to very low coefficient of friction, good wettability, extreme hardness and good biocompatibility. The wear particles are less bioactive as well. The fundamental problem of a ceramic bearing surface is its intrinsic brittleness. The previous generations of C on C bearing exhibited higher fracture rates and thus the fourth generation (Delta Ceramic) of ceramic was developed to prevent this complication. Delta ceramic is an Alumina Matrix Composition (AMC) (74% Al, 25% Zr, 0.5% SrO, and 0.5% CrO2) where the ceramic microstructure is designed to prevent crack initiation and propagation. One complication that could be of potential concern is squeaking. Squeaking is a unique complication noted mostly in C on C bearing. The reported percentage in the literature ranges from 1 to 20% [9, 10]. The exact cause of squeaking is unknown but a multifactorial etiology is the most likely cause. Some of the reasons attributed are malposition and edge loading, micro separation and subluxation of the femoral head [11], disruption of fluid film lubrication leading to stripe wear [11], component malposition leading to edge loading [12] and short femoral neck. Majority of patients notice it during some activity like stair climbing, walking and do not complain about it but some can be bothered by the noise without any functional deficit. Stryker Accolade stem was noted to have higher incidence of squeaking than other implants [13]. Recently a new design called the "delta motion" has been introduced, which essentially is a blended delta ceramic on a titanium alloy mono block acetabular shell and a large head ceramic on ceramic bearing. The advantage of this design is the stability offered by large head and decrease in the potential volumetric wear at the bearing surface. *One* theoretical concern is going to be the trunnion related problems with a large ceramic head and metal stem.

Metal on Metal (MoM) Bearing

The earliest MoM was attempted in the 1930's but was popularized by Mackee, Watson, Ring and Farfar in the 1950's. By mid-1970 the MoM had lost the battle of bearing surfaces and low friction arthroplasty of Metal on Polyethylene was the bearing of choice in clinical use. But, with aseptic loosening due to polyethylene particles and minimal wear in the MoM bearing there was a renewed interest in MoM bearing in the 1990's and early part of first decade of the 21st century. In the last couple of years there has been recognition in the problems of MoM bearing and largely has fallen out of favor with arthroplasty surgeons. The negative publicity associated with the dramatic failure of ASR (Articular Surface

Replacement) by Depuy has added to the disrepute of MoM bearing.

The advantage of MoM bearing has been its wear properties. It is bone conserving and also has the added advantage of using a larger head thus having a lesser chance for dislocation. But, complications which have been noted with this bearing surface have been called as Metallosis, Aseptic Lymphocytic- Vasculitis Associated Lesion (ALVAL), Adverse Reaction to Metal Debris (ARMD) and Pseudo tumors. Metallosis is the gross visual staining of tissues with metal debris while ALVAL is the histological finding which can be present even in the absence of any gross visual changes. Pseudo tumors are collection of metallic debris and tissue response to it with large cystic or fibrotic mass. Langton *et al.* have noted ARMD of 6% for large MoM THA at 41 month follow up which has further risen to 18% in a recent review [14]. Pseudo tumors could be essentially asymptomatic and have been noted to be present in about 4% of MoM hip replacements.

MoM bearings have very low tolerance for cup malposition and the optimum position recommended has been 45° of inclination and 20° anteversion. Higher inclination angle has been associated with significant edge loading and thus a greater chance of ARMD. The other problem with a MoM bearing is the relationship of component size and chances of revision, smaller the component greater the chance of revision and this has been attributed to poorer lubrication and reduced arc of motion. Cobalt (Co) and Chromium (Cr) ions have consistently measured to be higher in patients who have had metal on metal bearing surfaces. Though there is no exact cut off values which can define safety; presently, the consensus is that 2ng/ml is the cut off values for Co and Cr blood concentration [15].

Wear

Wear can be defined as damage to a solid surface, generally involving progressive loss of material due to relative motion between two interacting surfaces. Wear pattern is related to the physical nature of the interacting surfaces as well as the type of motion between the surfaces as well. Broadly, wear can be classified into 4 types though many are described:

• Adhesive Wear

- Abrasive Wear
- Fatigue Wear
- Corrosive Wear

Adhesive Wear

At inertia there is a static bond that forms between two interacting surfaces; if the temporary bond that forms between the surfaces are stronger than that of the material strength of one of the substrates then the weaker surface will lose material and line the stronger surface and the thin lining on the strong surface will form particles that are present in the movement interface.

Abrasive Wear

The surface of most materials has small peaks called as "Asperities" which can remove material from the counter surface in relative motion- that type of wear generation is called as abrasive wear.

Fatigue Wear

Fatigue is the mechanical loss of material strength due to repeated cyclical loading thus leading to initiation and propagation of cracks along the sliding or rolling surfaces.

Corrosive Wear

This mechanism involves all the mechanical processes of wear in combination with chemical reaction leading to damage to the surfaces.

Wear Modes

While we discussed the mechanism of wear in the previous section we will discuss the wear modes that occur in total hip arthroplasty. There are basically 4 modes in which wear occurs in THA. Mode 1 is at the primary articulation whereas type 2, 3, 4 occur at other modular junctions as a function of design or material property of the THA components (Fig. 5). Table 2 shows the common wear pattern and strategies to prevent wear or reduce its effect.

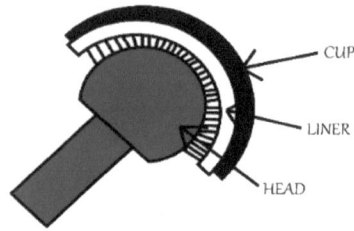

WEAQR OCCURS IN THE ARTICULAR SURFACE

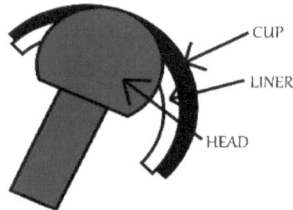

WEAR HAPPENS BETWEEN HEAD & THE METALIC CUP AFTER
WEARING THROUGH THE LINER

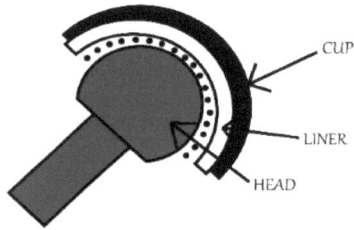

WEAR BECAUSE OF FOREIGN BODY BETWEEN THE HEAD & THE LINER

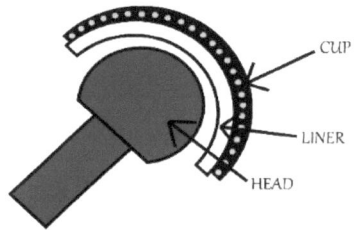

WEAR HAPPENS BETWEEN CUP AND THE LINER SURFACE

Fig. (5). Illustration of the various modes of wear.

Implant Selection During Total Hip Replacement

Early total hip designs were all cemented constructs and with minimal modularity.

With better understanding of orthophillic metallurgy, tribology and need for implant modularity there are a range of prosthetic options that have been developed. One of the unfortunate downside has been that the market has been flush with various designs of prosthesis and new iterant of the same design that it is hard to objectively compare the outcomes of various designs. In the last couple of decades there has been a changing trend with increased usage of uncemented components and decreased usage of cemented components.

Table 2. Wear modes and prevention strategies.

Wear Mode	Wear Interfaces	Prevention
Type 1	At the articular surface	• Improving the quality of polyethylene. • Hard on hard bearing has minimal type 1 wear • Highly Cross-linked poly has helped reduce type 1 wear
Type 2	Prosthetic head and the metal cup after wear through the acetabular liner	• Early recognition of liner damage and XLPE has helped reduce this wear pattern as well
Type 3	Wear due to presence of third body component in the articulating surfaces	• Intraoperative techniques to clear the cement, bone, ceramic and metallic debris by thorough lavage to prevent damage to the surfaces
Type 4	Occurs at the non-bearing secondary surface between the acetabular liner and the cup	• Improvement in the liner locking mechanisms will help decrease backside motion • Using mono-block blended acetabular components will eliminate backside wear altogether

The acetabular components have also tended to drift from cemented to the uncemented designs. The erroneous attribute of cement being the culprit in the wear process has largely contributed to this situation. The advantages of a cemented acetabular component is that it has equivalent to better survivorship than uncemented and cost effective but unfortunately the down sides are the inability to use alternate bearing surfaces. In the uncemented designs there is the advantage of using either a ceramic or metal bearing but has the problems of increased cost of components, back side wear in polyethylene liners and squeaking in ceramic liners. In a Swedish Hip Arthroplasty Registry (SHAR) evaluation of 1,70,413 total hip arthroplasty comparison of uncemented and cemented acetabular cups. Uncemented cup components had a higher risk of cup revision due to aseptic loosening (RR = 1.8, Cl: 1.6–2.0), whereas uncemented stem components had a lower risk of stem revision due to aseptic loosening (RR = 0.4, CI: 0.3–0.5) when compared to cemented components [14]. In a meta-analysis by Toossi *et al.* looking at acetabular component survivorship with at least 10 year follow up showed that the odds ratio for survivorship of a cemented acetabular component to be 1.60 (95% confidence interval, 1.32 to 2.40; p = 0.002) when adjustments for factors including age, sex, and mean duration of follow-up were made. In their study they do mention of the limitations of their study such as statistical method used and importantly the new generation of uncemented cups are a vast improvement over the previous generation of cups but having said that they concluded that there was no evidence that uncemented cups have done better than the cemented cups and in fact survivorship was better with cemented cups [15].

The stem options in total hip replacement have expanded in the recent decades with the advent of multiple un-cemented stem options. Still, the fundamental options in femoral stems are the cemented and un-cemented stems. The cemented mono block stem design originated with Dr. John Charnley and still remains one of the attractive options, though with some modifications. The advantages of the cemented stem is the low cost, great long term survivorship, minimal stress shielding of the proximal femur and intra operative flexibility to alter the version and limb length. The disadvantage of the cemented design is poor outcome in revision surgeries, hypotension during cementation sometimes leading to fatal complications and some increase in operative time.

The cemented stems work broadly on two philosophies- "taper slip principle" and "composite beam principle" (Fig. **6**). The taper slip principle works with a highly polished stainless steel or cobalt chrome stem. Even after cementation there is no tight interface between the stem and the cement mantle and thus with gait there is mild 1-2 mm movement at that interface leading to circumferential hoop stresses to be transmitted to the bone and thus maintaining bone strength. Exeter stem works on this principle and has excellent long term survivorship.

The composite beam principle works when the surface of the stem is roughened and there is a firm inter-digitation of cement with both the cancellous bone and the stem. Here the entire construct is rigid and generally stems following this principle have a collar which rests on the calcar.

Charnley   ## Exeter

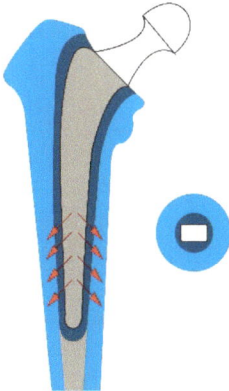

- Works on composite beam
- Implant+Cement+Bone work without interfacial movement
- Rough surface

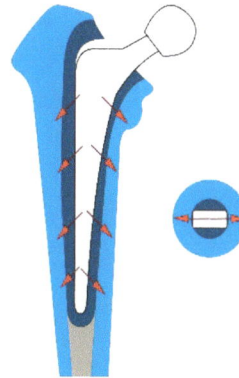

- Works on taper slip principle
- Bone+cement- Implant movement happens at the implant cement interface
- Highly polished surface

Fig. (6). Illustration depicting the principles of cemented stem fixation.

Table 3. Stem design types, practical utility and their clinical outcome.

Type	Stem Design	Fixation Location and Example	Survivorship Studies	Ideal Clinical Scenario
1	Single wedge	Metaphyseal Zimmer- ML taper Stryker- Accolade Depuy- corail stem		Primary THA Especially useful in direct anterior THA
2	Double wedge, metaphyseal filling	Metaphyseal Stryker- Secure fit Smith and Nephew- Synergy stem		Primary THA
3A	Tapered round	Metadiaphyseal Zimmer- FMT stem		Primary THA Revision THA with paprosky Type 2 defect
3B	Tapered splined	Metadiaphyseal Zimmer- Wagner cone prosthesis	92% Survivorship in 99 revisions with tapered fluted stems at 10 years by Bircher *et al.* [17]	Primary THA Revision THA with Paprosky Type 2 defect

(Table 3) contd.....

Type	Stem Design	Fixation Location and Example	Survivorship Studies	Ideal Clinical Scenario
3C	Tapered rectangular	Metadiaphyseal Zimmer- Alloclassic zweymuller stem Smith and Nephew- SL Stem		Primary THA Revision THA with Paprosky Type 2 defect
4	Fully coated cylindrical	Diaphyseal Depuy- AML stem	3.5% Revision for loosening at mean 14.2 yr. follow up in 170 hips of AML design by Weeden *et al.* [18]	Revision THA- Paprosky type 3A &3B defects Associated with proximal stress shielding Difficult to revise the stems
5	Modular	Diaphyseal Depuy- SROM system		Primary THA in special scenarios like DDH, Sequelae of Perthes, SCFE Revision THA with Paprosky Type 3 defects
6	Anatomical	Metaphyseal Stryker- Short Citation stem		Primary THA

Uncemented stems have seen tremendous improvement in design as well as fixation surfaces in the last two decades. Khanuja *et al.* [16] have classified the stems into six categories and have looked at their performance (Fig. **7**). Stems in Type 1 to 5 have a good track record with long term survivorship of 95% at 15-20 years in most designs (Table **3**). The early generation anatomical stems have had poor track record and have not done well esp. the cobalt-chromium design stems meanwhile the new generation Titanium stems have done well and their medium term survivorship has been encouraging.

Role of Large Femoral Heads in THA

The usage of large femoral heads has allowed significant improvement in hip stability as shown by various clinical data.

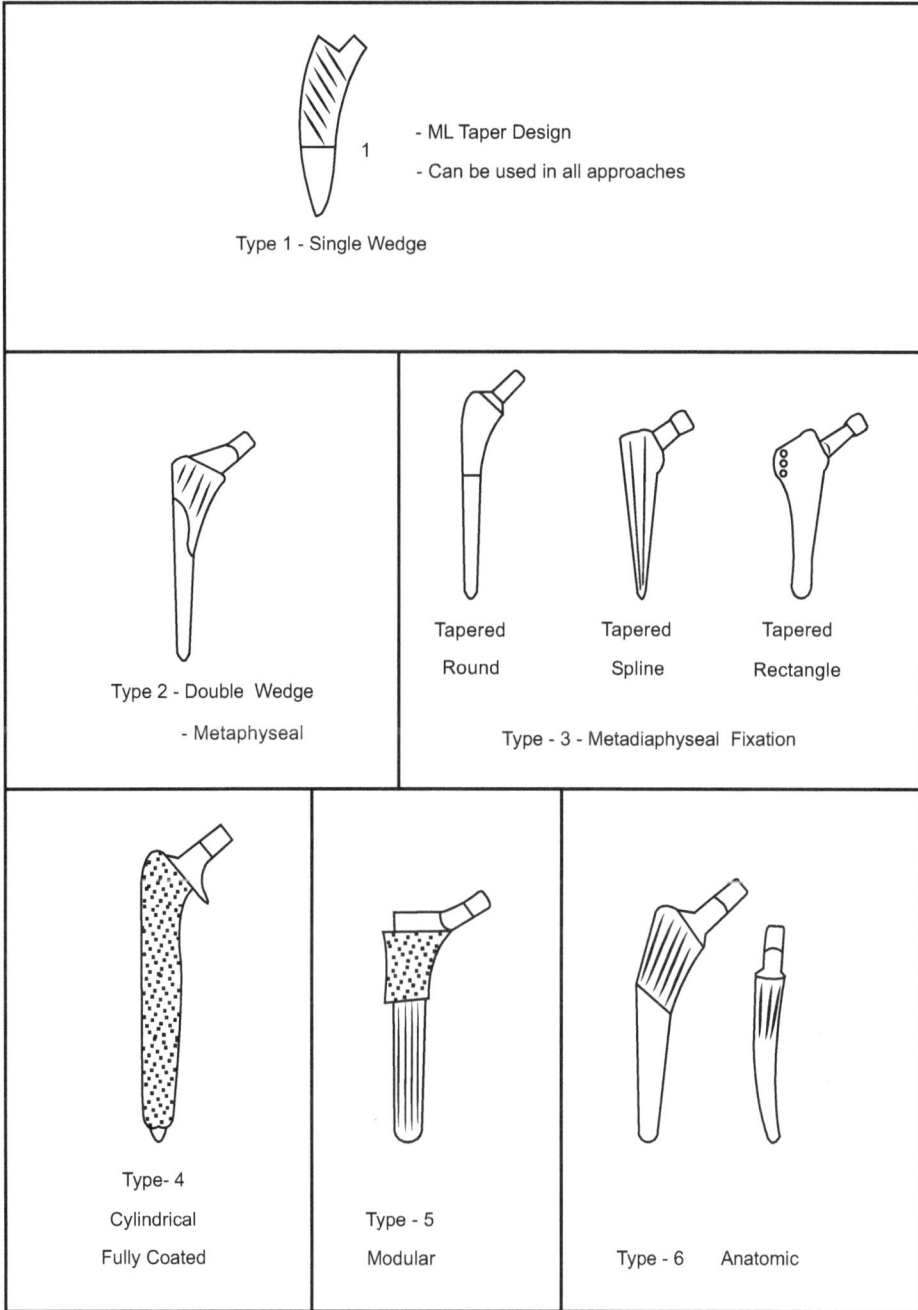

Fig. (7). Illustration showing various un-cemented stem design options.

Jump distance (JD) is the amount of translation that is required for the head to come out of the acetabular socket piece. The jump distance increases as the size of the femoral head increases. But, it is critical that the component is placed well in the acetabular socket piece. JD is also determined by the position of the acetabular cup with which has an inverse relationship for example increase in the abduction angle for a 32 mm head by 1 degree decreases the JD by 0.25 mm. In a study in the Norwegian Arthroplasty Registry [19] looking at 42,987 Primary THA there was a decrease in the revision rate for instability as the size of the femoral head increased from 28 mm to 32 mm. Similarly in a Mayo clinic registry study published in 2005, they looked at dislocation rates with the size of the femoral head in a cohort of 21,047 patients and found that with 32 mm heads the risk of dislocation was lowest and increased with 28 mm and was highest with 22 mm head.

Range of Motion (ROM) is another important factor which has been attributed to large femoral heads. More than the size of the head of femur it is the head neck ratio that determines the ROM. Ideally the head neck ratio of >2 will give a good ROM. The neck geometry as well as usage of skirting will also determine the ROM with trapezoidal neck and non-skirted heads giving the best stability [20].

With the increase of the head size beyond 36 mm there is not much improvement in the dislocation rates but volumetric wear becomes a serious concern. Schmalzried *et al.* have looked at retrieved THA bearings and found that with every mm increase in the size of the femoral head there is an increase of 6.3 mm/year of polyethylene wear [21]. Similarly, in a publication by Lachiewicz *et al.* cautioned against routine use of large femoral head in patients who have low index of suspicion for dislocation as the long term effects of increased volumetric wear is not well known [22]. It is safe to conclude that with the present available evidence 36 mm size should suffice for most clinical situation where there is an increased risk of dislocation with highly cross linked polyethylene as a bearing surface.

Recent Advances in Total Hip Arthroplasty

There has been a lot of interest of late on short stay total hip and knee arthroplasty. There are many reasons for this spurt in interest advances in pain management protocol, small incision surgeries, cost effectiveness of short stay for all involved and patients desire to return to their home and work life sooner than later. The short stay THA has reached a stage where certain dedicated centers in the US and other countries are trying day care total hip arthroplasty. "Short stay' and "accelerated Rehabilitation protocol" includes selecting a subset of patients who are highly motivated and pre-surgical counselling done, performing the surgery through either a mini posterior or direct anterior approach, using multi modal pain management protocol and starting post-operative physical therapy immediately on the day of surgery and progressing them quickly for discharge. In a study by Berger *et al.* using the minimally invasive technique of 100 consecutive patients 97% patients met all the inpatient Physical therapy goals required for discharge to home on the day of surgery. Outpatient therapy was initiated in 9% patients immediately and 62% by 1 week and all patients by 2 weeks [23].

Complications Following Total Hip Replacement

Total hip arthroplasty even though is described as "the operation of the century" by Lancet in 2007 it can be associated with significant complications [24]. Table below summarizes some of the important complications associated with this procedure (Table **4**).

Table 4. Important complications after THA.

General		Local	
Myocardial Infarction	0.5%	Leg Length Discrepancy as perceived by patient	30%
Symptomatic PE	0.5%	Infection	1.08%
Symptomatic DVT	1.3%	Dislocation	0.5-5%

Deep Vein Thrombosis (DVT) and Pulmonary Embolism (PE)

DVT is a potentially serious complication after THA especially if it becomes a PE and could have fatal or significant morbidity associated with it. Without some form of prophylaxis the incidence has been reported to be as high as 70% [25]. The high risk of DVT has been the foundation on which the recommendations for

DVT prophylaxis have been based. There are various prophylaxis regimens that have been advocated and there are a lot of variations to choose from. There have been recommendations which range from usage of pneumatic compression devices, Warfarin, unfractionated Heparin, Low Molecular Weight Heparin and Aspirin in various studies (Table **5**). The significant problem with the prophylaxis regime is higher incidence of bleeding complications and infection.

Table 5. Drugs available in the treatment of DVT.

Drug	Mechanism of Action	Advantages	Disadvantages
Heparin	Binds ATIII and leads to ternary complex which binds Thrombin, IXa and Xa	Short Half-life & easily reversed with Protamine sulfate No need to adjust in Renal failure	Unpredictable dose response Fixed dosage not to be used in DVT prophylaxis Parenteral administration required
LMWH	Selectively inhibit Xa but not thrombin	Fixed dosage once or twice daily	Only partially reversible with protamine Dosage adjustment in renal failure Parenteral administration require
Warfarin	Inhibits the Vit-K dependent factors like II, VII, IX and X	Oral dosing	Needs regular monitoring of PT/INR
Aspirin	Inhibits COX and decreases platelet aggregation by blocking production of Thromboxane A2	Oral dosing	Not as effective as other agents
Fondaparinux	Selectively inhibits factor Xa	Once daily dosing	Irreversible action Parenteral administration
Rivaroxaban	Direct inhibitor of factor Xa	Good Oral bioavailability	Irreversible action

Unique Points to Note for DVT Prophylaxis

Heparin

- Is administered with an APTT of 1-5 sec more than hospital upper normal
- Standard low dose heparin (5000U SC BID) is not recommended because it is ineffective

Low Molecular Weight Heparin

• Binds less to plasma proteins and can be used in fixed dosing

The latest American College of Chest Physician (ACCP) guidelines recommends that patients who undergo either a total hip arthroplasty (THA) or total knee arthroplasty (TKA), use of one of the following for a minimum of 10 to 14 days rather than no antithrombotic prophylaxis: low-molecular-weight heparin (LMWH), fondaparinux, apixaban, dabigatran, rivaroxaban, low-dose unfractionated heparin (LDUH), adjusted-dose vitamin K antagonist (VKA), aspirin [26]. They also suggested that the timing should be either 12 or more hours preoperatively/postoperatively than 4 or more hours preoperatively or postoperatively.

The problem with the guidelines is the confusion with the societies that prescribe them and even with the previous iteration of the same guidelines. The previous ACCP guidelines had recommended against using Aspirin for DVT prophylaxis but the present one permits the usage of aspirin as a single agent. American Academy of Orthopedic Surgery (AAOS) does recommend that patients who are not at high risk for bleeding should receive chemical as well as mechanical anti DVT measures but does not have a clear recommendation for patients with increased risk of bleeding and advises individualization of prophylaxis [27].

Dislocation

Dislocation after a primary THA varies in range from 0.2% to 7% [28].The dislocation rate is determined primarily by 3 factors- Patient related, surgeon related and surgery related. Majority of dislocations (up to 70%) happen in the first 6 weeks.

Patient related risk factors for dislocation are etiology and neuromuscular control. If a patient has a THA for a fracture etiology then the incidence of dislocation is higher than for arthritis and the possible explanation is that the capsule has not hypertrophied in a Neck of Femur fracture as it does in arthritis [29]. The overall dislocation rates after THA for NOF fractures are 6% and anterolateral approach has a lower dislocation rate than the posterolateral approach (2% *vs* 12%) [30].

Patients with neurological problems like Parkinson's disease and cerebral palsy have a higher dislocation rate.

The surgeon and surgery related risk factors are the surgical approach chosen, component placement and restoration of soft tissue tension. Table **6** looks at the various surgical approaches and associated incidences of dislocation. Early techniques of posterior THA was associated with high rates of dislocation but with the advent of meticulous posterior soft tissue repair the incidence of dislocation has come down to comparable levels. The recent interest in the direct anterior approach for THA has been to improve early functional outcome and reduction in the length of stay.

Table 6. Surmises various studies according to approaches and their dislocation rates.

Study	No. of Patients	Approach	Dislocation Percentage
Woo and Morrey *et al.* [31]	2459	Transtrochanteric -1241 Posterior -588 Anterolateral -660	2.2% 5.6% 2.2%
Vicar and Coleman *et al.* [32]	269	Transtrochanteric-136 Posterior -42 Anterolateral - 91	2.2% 9.5% 2.2%
Masonis *et al.* [33]	13,203	Transtrochanteric-2988 Posterior -3719 Anterolateral -826 Posterior(repair) -2262	1.27% 3.95% 2.18% 2.03%
Pellici *et al.** [34]	1074	Posterior -555 Posterior(repair) -519	4.68% 0.2%

Pellici *et al.* - Compares the posterior approach where a complete posterior soft tissue repair was done with that of a technique with no repair.

Soft tissue tension plays a critical role in stability of the hip joint. Restoration of the offset helps in reduction of the dislocation rate [35]. The trans-trochanteric approach with trochanteric non-union and trochanteric escape of more than 1 cm is associated with a six fold increase in dislocation rate [31]. Component position has a very important role to play in the stability of the THA; appropriate amount of anteversion in the acetabular cup at 20 ± 10 degree and abduction of 40 ± 10 degree is critical in reducing the incidence of dislocation. Lewinnick *et al.* [36] described that the position within the above "safe zone" is the best position to prevent dislocation.

Recent Developments in THA

Short Stem Hip Arthroplasty

Uncemented THA has evolved tremendously over the last couple of decades but still certain problems remain like optimal load transfer to the proximal femur, proximal and distal stem dimension mismatch, minimal damage during revision and ability to perform THA through minimally invasive approaches. To address these issues one of the approach advocated is the short stem THA. Technically short stem implants have been defined as ones <120 mm in length which is generally at the meta-diaphyseal junction [37]. The reported advantages of the short stem are it is bone preserving and soft tissue sparing, optimal loading of the proximal metaphysis and prevents stress shielding [38], absence of thigh pain as there is no diaphyseal contact of metal [16], easy to use in minimally invasive approaches as well as revision as it does not need extensive dissection.

Modification of surgical technique is important with these implants- Head neck resection to be conservative and medially the cut should start at the head neck junction. The other common problem with this stem design is a Varus malposition as there is no diaphyseal centering of the stem.

Table 7. Short stem design and survivorship in various studies.

Study	No. of Hips	Stem Design	Mean Follow-up	Survivorship
Falez *et al.* [39]	160	Mayo	4.7 years	97.5%
Santori *et al.* [40]	129	Custom design	8 years	100%
Lombardi *et al.* [41]	650	Taperloc microplasty stem Biomet	2 years	99.6%
Patel *et al.* [42]	65	Short Citation stem from Stryker	2 years	100%
Kim and Oh [43]	256	IPS stem from Depuy	5.6 years	99.7%

Outcomes and survivorship of the short stem is shown in Table **7**. Short stems are evolving and the data of their usage is limited in comparison to the vast amount on other designs. This design is not fit for patients who are osteoporotic as it can lead it inadequate primary metaphyseal stability. Most series report minimal to no thigh pain in their series with a peri-prosthetic fracture rate that ranges from 0 to 5.7% [40]. Some series have reported high rates of malposition of up to 68.2% typically in Varus which indicates a learning curve to this procedure [44].

Navigation in Total Hip Arthroplasty

The optimal acetabular cup position is important to avoid impingement which can lead to dislocation, accelerated wear and pain [45]. The optimum implant positioning is aided by mechanical alignment guides, intra-operative anatomical landmarks. Combined anteversion of the hip is critical in determining the outcome after THA which has been described as $25\text{-}45^0$ in men and $30\text{-}45^0$ in women [46]. DiGioia *et al.* showed in 1998 for the first time the application of computer navigation to improve the outcome of component positioning in THA [47]. Computer assisted hip replacement can be an active or a passive system; the active system consists of using a robotic arm assist in cup placement while the passive system has two variations-image based or imageless system. An image based systems where pre-surgical CT scanning is done and used as a reference for cup placement or an imageless system uses a virtual model with infra-red trackers to get optimal cup positioning. The limitation in the navigation system is the accurate acquisition of the anterior frontal plane which involves accurate recording of the anterior superior iliac spine and the pubic tubercle.

Conventional cup placement could result in outliers in almost 50% of the cases as shown by Kalteis *et al.* [48]. Navigation system helps to improve the cup placement in the safe zone in 87% for inclination and 79% for flexion and 73% for combination of inclination and flexion [49]. Navigation is an expensive technology and would definitely help in improvement of cup positioning in THA; its wide adaptability would depend on the cost of technology, ease of use and training of surgeons in its usage.

Minimally Invasive (MIS) Total Hip Arthroplasty

Many surgeons have attempted to reduce the length of incision, tissue trauma during the performance of THA. There is no consensus on the length of incision to be termed as MIS for THA but generally the accepted length of incision is 6-10 cm. The approaches have also varied from anterior, antero-lateral, postero-lateral, direct lateral and a direct 2 incision surgery. The advocates of MIS THA claim that it reduces soft tissue trauma, less post-operative pain and reduces length of stay and the detractors of MIS criticize it because there is reduced visualization leading to component mal-position, implant loosening and increased incidence of neurovascular damage [50]. In a meta-analysis by Cheng T *et al.* looking into 12 studies pooled data the incidence of dislocation, transient nerve palsy and infection was more common in MIS rather than standard Incision (SI) THA [51]. The general consensus regarding MIS THA is that it has a steep learning curve and patients have to be carefully selected excluding obese or with coxa profunda picture.

Our Approach to THA

Our approach has been refined over a period of time based on experience and convenience. We use a standard posterior approach with meticulous posterior soft tissue repair in most patients. In a thin, lean patient we use a direct anterior approach for our primary THA. Most of our revisions are carried out through a Posterior approach. Our implant selection is dictated by patient factors and if it is a primary or revision scenario. Our primary implant of choice is an uncemented THA with a metaphyseal canal filling stem design and an uncemented cup. We use a highly polished stem if there is a Dorr type C canal or patient desires an affordable choice.

Given the present alternatives available, the possible need for life long surveillance with blood ion levels, the medicolegal problems with a metal on metal bearing it is safe to conclude that a surgeon has to be highly selective and have a detailed discussion with their patient before embarking on a metal on metal bearing surface. We do not offer the MoM bearing to our patients routinely and have rarely ever needed to perform a MoM in our practice currently.

Our bearing surface of choice is metal on highly cross linked polyethylene and occasionally in young individuals we use a ceramic on ceramic bearing. All our patients are mobilized the day after surgery and would follow hip precautions for the first 6 weeks. In house DVT prophylaxis with LMWH is given for 4-5 days and transitioned to oral Aspirin for 35 days duration on out-patient therapy.

Our Peri-operative Pain Management Protocol

We have a streamlined protocol for the post-operative pain management.

Our Pain medication protocol includes that all patients receive IV Paracetamol (PCT) 1 gm three times a day for 3 days and later given on PRN basis. The patients are also prescribed Oral Low dose tramadol and Paracetamol combination (37.5 mg and 325 mg respectively) so that a maximum of 4 grams of PCT is administered in a day along with 75 mg of Pregabalin to address the neuropathic component of pain. We also use NSAID's as tolerated if the patient's renal functions are normal on a PRN basis. The next step is to institute a buprenorphine patch if patient has pain. We start either with a 5 mcg or 10 mcg patch and monitor the patient's pain tolerance. In spite of all the measures if the patient does not find relief of pain then parenteral IV morphine/fentanyl is administered by a dedicated team of anesthetist. Empirically, the need for parenteral opioids in our practice has been less than 10% and most of them are comfortable with our above regime. We do not follow peri-capsular injections as a couple of patients in the past have had early postoperative infections and the hospital infection control team found that one of the potential sources of contamination has been the multiple vials needed to make the cocktail injections. Still, we find merit in peri-capsular injections and are exploring safe ways to have the peri-capsular injections prepared.

CONFLICT OF INTEREST

The authors confirm that the authors have no conflict of interest to declare for this publication.

ACKNOWLEDGEMENTS

Declared none.

REFERENCES

[1]   Schutzer SF, Harris WH. Trochanteric osteotomy for revision total hip arthroplasty. 97% union rate using a comprehensive approach. Clin Orthop Relat Res 1988; 2227: 172-83.

[2]   Huffman GR, Ries MD. Combined vertical and horizontal cable fixation of an extended trochanteric osteotomy site. J Bone Joint Surg Am 2003; 85-A(2): 273-7.

[PMID: 12571305]

[3]   Jones LC, Hungerford DS. Cement disease. Clin Orthop Relat Res 1987; (225): 192-206.
        [PMID: 3315375]

[4]   Amstutz HC, Campbell P, Kossovsky N, Clarke IC. Mechanism and clinical significance of wear
        debris-induced osteolysis. Clin Orthop Relat Res 1992; (276): 7-18.
        [PMID: 1537177]

[5]   Beksaç B, Salas A, González Della Valle A, Salvati EA. Wear is reduced in THA performed with
        highly cross-linked polyethylene. Clin Orthop Relat Res 2009; 467(7): 1765-72.
        [http://dx.doi.org/10.1007/s11999-008-0661-1] [PMID: 19082863]

[6]   Dorr LD, Wan Z, Shahrdar C, Sirianni L, Boutary M, Yun A. Clinical performance of a Durasul highly
        cross-linked polyethylene acetabular liner for total hip arthroplasty at five years. J Bone Joint Surg Am
        2005; 87(8): 1816-21.
        [http://dx.doi.org/10.2106/JBJS.D.01915] [PMID: 16085624]

[7]   Manley MT, Capello WN, Bierbaum BE, Ramakrishnan R, Naughton M, Sutton K. Five-year
        experience with Crossfire highly cross-linked polyethylene. Clin Orthop Relat Res 2005; (441): 143-
        50.

[8]   Kurtz SM, Gawel HA, Patel JD. History and systematic review of wear and osteolysis outcomes for
        first-generation highly crosslinked polyethylene. Clin Orthop Relat Res 2011; 469(8): 2262-77.
        [http://dx.doi.org/10.1007/s11999-011-1872-4] [PMID: 21431461]

[9]   Capello WN. D 'Antonio JA, Manley MT. Alumina-on-alumina bearings in total hip arthroplasty:
        clinical results, osteolysis, breakage, and noise. J Arthroplasty 2007; 22: 311-1.
        [http://dx.doi.org/10.1016/j.arth.2006.12.076]

[10]   Jarrett CA, Ranawat A, Bruzzone M, Rodriguez J, Ranawat C. The squeaking hip: an underreported
        phenomenon of ceramic-on ceramic total hip arthroplasty. J Arthroplasty 2007; 22: 302.
        [http://dx.doi.org/10.1016/j.arth.2006.12.012]

[11]   Ranawat AS, Ranawat CS. The squeaking hip: a cause for concern-agrees. Orthopedics 2007; 30(9):
        738-43.

[12]   Walter WL, Otoole GC, Walter WK, Ellis A, Zicat BA. Squeaking in ceramic-on-ceramic hips: the
        importance of acetabular component orientation. J Arthroplasty 2007; 22(4): 496-503.
        [http://dx.doi.org/10.1016/j.arth.2006.06.018] [PMID: 17562404]

[13]   Scott S, Capozzi JD. Squeaking in third- and fourth-generation ceramic-on-ceramic total hip
        arthroplasty. Meta-analysis and systematic review. J Arthroplasty 2011; 0: 1-9.

[14]   Hailer NP, Garellick G, Karrholm J. Uncemented and cemented primary total hip arthroplasty in the
        Swedish Hip Arthroplasty Register. Acta Orthopaedica 2010; 81(1): 34-41.

[15]   Toossi N, Adeli B, Timperley AJ, Haddad FS, Maltenfort M, Parvizi J. Acetabular components in total
        hip arthroplasty: Is there evidence that cementless fixation is better? J Bone Joint Surg Am 2013; 95:
        168-74.

[16]   Khanuja HS, Vakil JJ, Goddard MS, Mont MA. Cementless femoral fixation in total hip arthroplasty. J
        Bone Joint Surg Am 2011; 93(5): 500-9.
        [http://dx.doi.org/10.2106/JBJS.J.00774] [PMID: 21368083]

[17]   Bircher HP, Riede U, Lüem M, Ochsner PE. The value of the Wagner SL revision prosthesis for bridging large femoral defects. Orthopade 2001; 30(5): 294-303.
[http://dx.doi.org/10.1007/s001320050611] [PMID: 11417237]

[18]   Weeden SH, Paprosky WG. Minimal 11-year follow-up of extensively porous-coated stems in femoral revision total hip arthroplasty. J Arthroplasty 2002; 17(4) (Suppl. 1): 134-7.
[http://dx.doi.org/10.1054/arth.2002.32461] [PMID: 12068424]

[19]   Byström S, Espehaug B, Furnes O, Havelin LI. Femoral head size is a risk factor for total hip luxation: a study of 42,987 primary hip arthroplasties from the Norwegian Arthroplasty Register. Acta Orthop Scand 2003; 74(5): 514-24.
[http://dx.doi.org/10.1080/00016470310017893] [PMID: 14620970]

[20]   Rathi P, Pereira GC, Giordani M, Di Cesare PE. The pros and cons of using larger femoral heads in total hip arthroplasty. Am J Orthop 2013; 42(8): E53-9.
[PMID: 24078959]

[21]   Schmalzried TP, Callaghan JJ. Wear in total hip and knee replacements. J Bone Joint Surg Am 1999; 81(1): 115-36.
[PMID: 9973062]

[22]   Lachiewicz PF, Heckman DS, Soileau ES, Mangla J, Martell JM. Femoral head size and wear of highly cross-linked polyethylene at 5 to 8 years. Clin Orthop Relat Res 2009; 467(12): 3290-6.
[http://dx.doi.org/10.1007/s11999-009-1038-9] [PMID: 19690932]

[23]   Berger RA, Jacobs JJ, Meneghini RM, Della Valle C, Paprosky W, Rosenberg AG. Rapid rehabilitation and recovery with minimally invasive total hip arthroplasty. Clin Orthop Relat Res 2004; (429): 239-47.
[http://dx.doi.org/10.1097/01.blo.0000150127.80647.80] [PMID: 15577494]

[24]   Learmonth ID, Young C, Rorabeck C. The operation of the century: total hip replacement. Lancet 2007; 370(9597): 1508-19.
[http://dx.doi.org/10.1016/S0140-6736(07)60457-7] [PMID: 17964352]

[25]   Kim YH, Oh SH, Kim JS. Incidence and natural history of deep-vein thrombosis after total hip arthroplasty. A prospective and randomised clinical study. J Bone Joint Surg Br 2003; 85(5): 661-5.
[PMID: 12892186]

[26]   Prevention of VTE in orthopedic surgery patients: antithrombotic therapy and prevention of thrombosis. American College of Chest Physicians evidence-based clinical practice guidelines Chest 2012; 141(2 Suppl): e278S-325S.

[27]   American Academy of Orthopaedic Surgeons clinical practice guideline on preventing venous thromboembolic disease in patients undergoing elective hip and knee arthroplasty. American Academy of Orthopaedic Surgeons clinical practice guideline on preventing venous thromboembolic disease in patients undergoing elective hip and knee arthroplasty. Rosemont (IL): American Academy of Orthopaedic Surgeons (AAOS) 211; 824.

[28]   Patel PD, Potts A, Froimson MI. The dislocating hip arthroplasty: prevention and treatment. J Arthroplasty 2007; 22(4) (Suppl. 1): 86-90.
[http://dx.doi.org/10.1016/j.arth.2006.12.111] [PMID: 17570285]

[29]   Lee BP, Berry DJ, Harmsen WS, Sim FH. Total hip arthroplasty for the treatment of an acute fracture of the femoral neck: long-term results. J Bone Joint Surg Am 1998; 80(1): 70-5.
[PMID: 9469311]

[30]   Enocson A, Hedbeck CJ, Tidermark J, Pettersson H, Ponzer S, Lapidus LJ. Dislocation of total hip replacement in patients with fractures of the femoral neck. Acta Orthop 2009; 80(2): 184-9.
[http://dx.doi.org/10.3109/17453670902930024] [PMID: 19404800]

[31]   Woo RY, Morrey BF. Dislocations after total hip arthroplasty. J Bone Joint Surg Am 1982; 64(9): 1295-306.
[PMID: 7142237]

[32]   Vicar AJ, Coleman CR. A comparison of the anterolateral, transtrochanteric, and posterior surgical approaches in primary total hip arthroplasty. Clin Orthop Relat Res 1984; (188): 152-9.
[PMID: 6467710]

[33]   Masonis JL, Bourne RB. Surgical approach, abductor function, and total hip arthroplasty dislocation. Clin Orthop Relat Res 2002; (405): 46-53.
[http://dx.doi.org/10.1097/00003086-200212000-00006] [PMID: 12461355]

[34]   Pellicci PM, Bostrom M, Poss R. Posterior approach to total hip replacement using enhanced posterior soft tissue repair. Clin Orthop Relat Res 1998; (355): 224-8.
[http://dx.doi.org/10.1097/00003086-199810000-00023] [PMID: 9917607]

[35]   Fackler CD, Poss R. Dislocation in total hip arthroplasties. Clin Orthop Relat Res 1980; (151): 169-78.
[PMID: 7418301]

[36]   Lewinnek GE, Lewis JL, Tarr R, Compere CL, Zimmerman JR. Dislocations after total hip-replacement arthroplasties. J Bone Joint Surg Am 1978; 60(2): 217-20.
[PMID: 641088]

[37]   McTighe T, Stulberg SD, Keppler L, *et al.* A classification system for short uncemented total hip arthroplasty. Bone Joint J 2013; 95-B (Suppl.): 260.

[38]   Pipino F. The bone-prosthesis interaction. J Orthop Traumatol 2000; 1(1): 3-9.
[http://dx.doi.org/10.1007/PL00012193]

[39]   Falez F, Casella F, Panegrossi G, Favetti F, Barresi C. Perspectives on metaphyseal conservative stems. J Orthop Traumatol 2008; 9(1): 49-54.
[http://dx.doi.org/10.1007/s10195-008-0105-4] [PMID: 19384482]

[40]   Santori FS, Santori N. Mid-term results of a custom-made short proximal loading femoral component. J Bone Joint Surg Br 2010; 92(9): 1231-7.
[http://dx.doi.org/10.1302/0301-620X.92B9.24605] [PMID: 20798440]

[41]   Lombardi AV Jr, Berend KR, Ng VY. Stubby stems: good things come in small packages. Orthopedics 2011; 34(9): e464-6.
[PMID: 21902132]

[42]   Patel RM, Smith MC, Woodward CC, Stulberg SD. Stable fixation of short-stem femoral implants in patients 70 years and older. Clin Orthop Relat Res 2012; 470(2): 442-9.
[http://dx.doi.org/10.1007/s11999-011-2063-z] [PMID: 21927967]

[43] Kim YH, Oh JH. A comparison of a conventional *versus* a short, anatomical metaphyseal-fitting cementless femoral stem in the treatment of patients with a fracture of the femoral neck. J Bone Joint Surg Br 2012; 94(6): 774-81.
[http://dx.doi.org/10.1302/0301-620X.94B6.29152] [PMID: 22628591]

[44] Gilbert RE, Salehi-Bird S, Gallacher PD, Shaylor P. The Mayo Conservative Hip: experience from a district general hospital. Hip Int 2009; 19(3): 211-4.
[PMID: 19876874]

[45] Malik A, Maheshwari A, Dorr LD. Impingement with total hip replacement. J Bone Joint Surg Am 2007; 89(8): 1832-42.
[http://dx.doi.org/10.2106/JBJS.F.01313] [PMID: 17671025]

[46] Ranawat CS, Maynard MJ. Modern techniques of cemented total hip arthroplasty. Tech Orthop 1991; 6: 17-25.
[http://dx.doi.org/10.1097/00013611-199109000-00004]

[47] DiGioia AM, Jaramaz B, Blackwell M, *et al.* The Otto Aufranc Award. Image guided navigation system to measure intraoperatively acetabular implant alignment. Clin Orthop Relat Res 1998; (355): 8-22.
[PMID: 9917587]

[48] Kalteis T, Handel M, Herold T, Perlick L, Baethis H, Grifka J. Greater accuracy in positioning of the acetabular cup by using an image-free navigation system. Int Orthop 2005; 29(5): 272-6.
[http://dx.doi.org/10.1007/s00264-005-0671-5] [PMID: 16082540]

[49] Jenny JY, Boeri C, Dosch JC, Uscatu M, Ciobanu E. Navigated non-image-based positioning of the acetabulum during total hip replacement. Int Orthop 2009; 33(1): 83-7.
[http://dx.doi.org/10.1007/s00264-007-0479-6] [PMID: 18004568]

[50] Smith TO, Blake V, Hing CB. Minimally invasive *versus* conventional exposure for total hip arthroplasty: a systematic review and meta-analysis of clinical and radiological outcomes. Int Orthop 2011; 35(2): 173-84.
[http://dx.doi.org/10.1007/s00264-010-1075-8] [PMID: 20559827]

[51] Cheng T, Feng JG, Liu T, Zhang XL. Minimally invasive total hip arthroplasty: a systematic review. Int Orthop 2009; 33(6): 1473-81.
[http://dx.doi.org/10.1007/s00264-009-0743-z] [PMID: 19277652]

SUBJECT INDEX

www.ingramcontent.com/pod-product-compliance
Lightning Source LLC
Chambersburg PA
CBHW041728210326
41598CB00008B/810